family c

the FAT,
FIBRE and
CARBOHYDRATE
counter

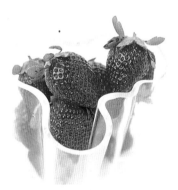

The publisher would like to thank the manufacturers who have contributed nutritional information about their products. Every care has been taken to ensure that all the information in this book was correct when the book went to press, however, some products may have been modified or discontinued since then, so check the labels for exact information. This book is not intended to replace professional medical advice and the publisher cannot be held liable for any action or claim arising from the use of this book.

MURDOCH BOOKS®

Sydney • London • Vancouver • New York

FINDING THE RIGHT BALANCE of food is important to the quality of our lives. In a balanced diet, the contribution of fat to total energy should not be more than 25–30%, and most of this should come from unsaturated, rather than saturated fats. Most energy should come from foods high in carbohydrates (60%) and a moderate amount from foods high in protein (15%).

If you are trying to lose weight, you must reduce your fat intake. However, this doesn't mean that fats should be removed from the diet altogether as they are essential to our health. One of their many functions is to provide a vehicle for the fat soluble vitamins A, D, E and K, and they also promote healthy blood, nerves, muscles and skin. Certain fats are also essential for children's growth.

However, a diet that is relatively low in fat is important for everyone's good health. All fats should be eaten sparingly, but there are some that make healthier choices than others. The best choice is polyunsaturated and monounsaturated fats, which actually lower blood cholesterol levels and are found in fish, seeds, wholegrains, nuts, vegetable oils and margarines. Polyunsaturated fats are also a source of essential fatty acids known as omega-3 and omega-6 fats.

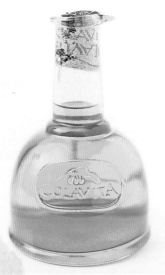

The type of fat to limit is saturated fat, which can raise cholesterol levels and may increase the risk of heart disease. Saturated fat is found in animal meats, full-cream dairy foods, butter and coconut and palm oil. To decrease your intake of saturated fats choose lean meats and trim all visible fat including chicken skin. Also, choose low-fat dairy products and polyunsaturated or monounsaturated oil and margarine, which may help lower cholesterol levels.

Fat turns up in the most unexpected places, so keep informed and read the fat content on labels. Fats carry flavour and are often added to processed foods to improve taste. Biscuits, pastries, cakes, chocolate, crisps, snack foods and take-away foods are a source of saturated fats.

Cholesterol is another type of fat, found in meat, shellfish, eggs, and dairy products. No plants contain cholesterol. Cholesterol intake should be monitored, but research has shown that it is more important to reduce saturated fat intake, which raises cholesterol than it is to reduce dietary cholesterol itself. When reading labels, remember that 'no cholesterol' does not mean 'no fat'.

Like the other fats, some cholesterol is necessary for a healthy body. We obtain cholesterol through animal foods, but the body also manufactures cholesterol in the liver. There are two different types of cholesterol called 'good' and 'bad' cholesterol. 'Bad' cholesterol is associated with an increased risk of heart disease and levels can grow when the diet is high in trans-fatty acids and saturated fats, and low in polyunsaturated and monounsaturated fats. On the other hand, 'good' cholesterol evels may be increased through exercise and a diet high in monounsaturated fats.

Dietary fibre is a very important part of our diet, and for most people the recommended intake is 30 grams per day. Fibre improves the health of the bowel, lowers cholesterol and reduces the risk of many diseases such as diabetes and colon cancer. It also promotes the feeling of a full stomach, which is valuable when dieting. To increase your fibre intake, limit processed foods and eat more carbohydrate-rich foods such as fresh fruit and vegetables, wholegrains and legumes. Nuts and seeds also provide fibre and should be included in your diet, although in smaller amounts if you are wishing to limit your fat content.

Carbohydrate foods are not only a source of dietary fibre, they are also an ideal source of fuel for the body. Of all the different kinds of foods, carbohydrates are the most easily converted to glucose and glycogen, which are the body's preferred energy sources. Excess carbohydrate, protein and even alcohol are not usually stored as body fat. It is only when we eat excess fat in our food, that our body stores it as body fat.

The distribution of body fat is important. Excess upper body fat creates the greatest health risk, in particular for coronary heart disease, high blood pressure and diabetes.

A balanced diet is easy if you follow some simple guidelines:

• Eat plenty of fresh fruit and vegetables, wholegrain breads and cereals and legumes, and drink about 5–6 glasses of water a day.

• Manage your saturated fat intake by trimming meats, choosing low-fat dairy products and avoiding fast foods, snack foods, pastries and deep-fried foods.

• Be aware of your intake of refined sugars, salt, alcohol, caffeine and additives, as you may wish to cut down or even eliminate these from your diet.

• Eat small amounts of fat from nuts, seeds, grains, fish, lean meats and vegetable oils.

• Eat adequate, but not excessive, amounts of protein from animal and plant sources.

Good health is not only dependent on a healthy diet, exercise is very important too. Exercise helps to increase vitality, raise

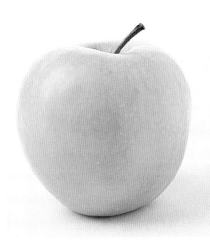

beneficial cholesterol levels and increase the metabolic rate, thereby making it easier to burn stored fat for fuel. For most people, the rush of everyday living is not enough to burn off excess fat in the diet, and the deficit gets stored as body fat. When exercise is combined with decreasing fat intake, exercise will use stored fat for energy. A healthy diet combined with regular exercise goes a long way to ensure a healthy body.

Body Mass Index (BMI) is an approximate way of calculating if you are in the healthy weight range. It is calculated as follows:

$$\frac{\text{weight (kg)}}{\text{height}^2 \text{ (m)}} = \text{BMI} \quad \text{e.g.} \quad \frac{72 \text{ kg}}{1.63^2 \text{ m}} = 27 \text{ BMI}$$

BMI criteria
Less than 20	underweight
20–25	healthy weight
25–30	overweight
over 30	obese

VITAMINS & MINERALS FUNCTIONS

Vitamin A

Promotes healthy eyes, skin and hair and also maintains the mucous membranes of the lungs and intestines. Improves immunity.

Beta Carotene

(can be converted by the body to Vitamin A)

One of the carotenoids—antioxidants that provide the yellow and orange colours in fresh produce. It improves immunity and protects against the effects of ageing and some cancers.

Vitamin B group

Provides energy. Important for normal function of the nervous and circulatory system. Needed for healthy skin, hair, nails and eyes.

Vitamin C

Produces collagen, which is needed for healthy skin, bones, cartilage and teeth. Improves stress response and helps the body to absorb iron.

Vitamin D

Needed to absorb calcium and phosphorus for healthy bones and teeth.

Vitamin E

Antioxidant. Needed for healthy circulation and healthy muscles, including the heart. Heals scar tissue.

Calcium

Maintains healthy bones and teeth. Regulates nerve and muscle function. Also needed for blood clotting.

Iron

Carries oxygen to the body cells via the blood.

Potassium

Maintains nerves, cells and muscles and promotes normal blood pressure and heartbeat.

Sodium

Needed for nerves and muscles and regulating the balance of fluid in the body.

Zinc

Needed for healthy eyes and skin and improves immunity. Essential for taste, smell and appetite. Maintains normal reproduction.

DEFICIENCY SIGNS	SOURCES
Eye, skin and hair problems, poor night vision, impaired bone growth and increased susceptibility to infections.	Liver, kidneys, fish liver oil, eggs, dairy foods, butter and margarine.
Increased susceptibility to infections.	Yellow, green, orange and red vegetables and fruit.
Anaemia, fatigue, nerve problems, decreased ability to cope with stress, depression, skin problems and greying hair.	Liver, kidneys, meat, poultry, fish, yeast, wholegrain breads and cereals, seeds, nuts, legumes, eggs, milk and leafy green vegetables.
Tissue breakdown, easy bleeding and bruising, fatigue, loss of appetite and depression.	Fruit and vegetables.
Muscle and bone weakness.	Egg yolk, cheese, margarine and oily fish (such as tuna, salmon and sardines), liver and oils.
Deficiency is rare. Prevents normal growth.	Egg yolks, meat, nuts, seeds, wholegrain cereals, wheatgerm, vegetable oils and margarine.
Rickets, osteoporosis, osteomalacia, cramps, muscle problems, high blood pressure and heart arrythmias.	Dairy products, almonds, brazil nuts, sardines, egg yolk, soya beans, brewer's yeast, carob, kelp, tofu and dried figs.
Fatigue, poor circulation, anaemia, dizziness, sore tongue and mouth ulcers.	Meat, chicken, fish, legumes, shellfish, nuts, wholegrain breads and cereals, eggs, molasses, leafy green vegetables and kelp.
Apathy, extreme thirst and fatigue.	Vegetables, fruit, avocadoes, wholegrain cereals, seeds, nuts, potatoes and pulses.
Deficiency is rare. Apathy, dehydration, vomiting, cramps.	Table salt, yeast extract, leg ham, sausages, bread, cheese, margarine and some take-away foods.
Decreased fertility and libido. Poor sense of taste and smell. Lack of appetite. Poor wound healing. Growth retardation and mental lethargy.	Meat, liver, eggs, seafood, legumes and wholegrain cereals.

GLOSSARY

ADDITIVES are chemicals added to food to preserve it, improve its appearance and palatability and to assist in its manufacture. Manufacturers are required by law to list additives on food labels and laws on their use are strict. A small number of people are intolerant of certain additives.

ANTIOXIDANTS protect against free radicals in the body, which are unstable chemicals that can promote heart disease, stroke or cancer. Our bodies produce their own antioxidants, but research has shown that certain vegetables, fruit, fish, nuts and seeds contain vitamins and minerals that also act as antioxidants to neutralize free radicals.

BASAL METABOLIC RATE is the minimum level of energy required to maintain all bodily functions, such as breathing, digestion and temperature. Some people have a high metabolic rate and can burn more kilojoules than other people. Exercise raises the metabolic rate by around 10%.

BLOOD PRESSURE is the pressure exerted by the blood on artery walls. High blood pressure is known as hypertension and is a factor in strokes, heart and kidney disease. Cutting back on salt and alcohol, learning how to combat stress, being physically active and maintaining a good body weight can all help lower blood pressure.

CARBOHYDRATES are the body's preferred source of fuel and should make up 50–60% of our diet. There are two types of carbohydrates:

Simple carbohydrates (or sugars) are found in fruit, some vegetables, honey and table sugar. Complex carbohydrates (or starch) are found in potatoes, cereals, bread, pasta and rice. Carbohydrates are broken down to glucose. When there is more glucose in the blood than the body immediately needs, the excess is converted into glycogen, which is stored in the liver and muscles as an energy reserve.

CHOLESTEROL is a type of fat found in all animals. 'Blood cholesterol' is manufactured in our liver, while 'dietary cholesterol' comes from eating any animal product. High cholesterol is a proven risk factor for coronary disease, and the best way to cut cholesterol levels is to cut saturated fat in the diet. Cholesterol is carried in the body attached to two lipoproteins, low-density (LDL) and high-density (HDL). HDL is known as the 'good cholesterol', and high levels reduce the risk of heart disease. High levels of the 'bad' cholesterol (LDL) do the reverse. Most people can lower their cholesterol levels by adopting a healthy lifestyle and diet, by being physically active and drinking alcohol in moderation.

DIABETES is characterised by a raised blood glucose level. This is due to an impairment in production, or decreased efficiency, of the hormone insulin, which takes glucose out of the blood and puts it into body cells where it is used for energy. There are two types of diabetes: Type 1, or Insulin Dependent Diabetes, needs insulin supplementation. Type 11, or Non-Insulin Dependent Diabetes, can be controlled through a diet high in complex carbohydrates and fibre, low in saturated fat. Regular physical activity and weight loss will also make a difference.

DIETARY FIBRE comes from plants and is digested in the large intestine during fermentation by bacteria. There are two types of fibre, insoluble and soluble, and most foods contain both. Fibre helps relieve constipation and conditions such as irritable bowel syndrome, and may also protect against bowel cancer and lower blood cholesterol. Cereals, fruit, vegetables, pulses, nuts and seeds are all good sources of fibre.

ELECTROLYTES are the mineral ions of sodium, potassium, calcium, magnesium and chloride. They are held in solution in body fluids and control much of the body's internal chemical reactions. Diarrhoea, vomiting and heavy sweating can disturb electrolyte balance.

ENERGY is needed by the body to perform physical work and also to run the body's internal functions. Energy is provided by carbohydrates, protein and fats in our food, and by alcohol. The energy value of food is measured in kilojoules (kJ). One calorie = 4.2 kJ.

ESSENTIAL FATTY ACIDS are part of the polyunsaturated fats group and are found in the omega-3 and omega-6 groups of fatty acids. They are essential to the body for growth and health and must be supplied from the diet. Omega-3 fats are found in salmon, tuna, sardines and mackerel, and in linseed, canola and soya oils. Omega-6 fats are found in sunflower, corn and safflower oils, and in soya beans, polyunsaturated margarine, walnuts and brazil nuts. Omega fats lower blood fat levels and protect the body from heart disease and stroke.

FREE RADICALS are unstable atoms in the body. Sometimes, in response to nicotine, UV rays and pollution, the body produces more free radicals than necessary. These may then react with cells to damage them and make them susceptible to cancers and other diseases. The body produces antioxidants to neutralize these free radicals, and eating plenty of fish, fruit and vegetables may also help.

HEART DISEASE has a number of risk factors, including high blood pressure and high blood cholesterol levels, often caused by a diet high in saturated fat, smoking, inactivity and obesity.

HYDROGENATED FATS are fats that have undergone a chemical alteration during processing. Hydrogenation adds hydrogen atoms to oils to form solid fats. The hydrogenation process can cause trans-fatty acids to form.

MINERALS are essential elements found in our food. They are necessary for the formation of body structure and for the regulation of all body processes.

MONOSODIUM GLUTAMATE (MSG) is used as a flavour enhancer in some processed foods and restaurants, particularly Chinese ones. It can cause allergic reactions such as headache, chest pain and asthma in MSG-sensitive people. You can avoid it in processed food by looking for 'flavour enhancer (621)' on labels.

MONOUNSATURATED FATS have one unsaturated double bond in their chemical structure. These fats may help to lower 'bad' cholesterol levels and raise 'good' cholesterol levels. They are found in large amounts in olive, canola, macadamia and peanut oils and nuts.

PRESERVATIVES are substances added to food to prevent it decomposing. The earliest preservatives were salt, vinegar and alcohol. Nowadays, artificial preservatives are also used, and some people are allergic to them. Frozen and canned food is usually free of preservatives because the method of packaging preserves the food.

POLYUNSATURATED FATS have two or more unsaturated double bonds in their chemical structure. They are found in fish and in vegetable oils. Polyunsaturated fats are the only source of the essential fatty acids, omega-3 and omega-6. Polyunsaturated fats help to lower 'bad' cholesterol levels and blood fat levels.

PHYTOESTROGENS are substances found in some plants that have a balancing effect on oestrogen levels. Phytoestrogens can be used when the body is either low or high in oestrogen. Soya beans are the best source of phytoestrogens. They are also found in legumes, sprouts, linseed, cabbage and corn.

PROTEINS are responsible for building and repairing new body tissues such as muscles, skin, hair, nails, blood cells, nerves and glands. They also form infection-fighting antibodies. Protein is a source of energy, and if more protein is consumed than the body needs, it can be stored as fat. Protein is divided into high-quality, such as in meat, eggs, fish and soya beans, and low-quality, such as in nuts, seeds, grains and legumes. Eating a mixture of proteins will provide enough quality protein, even for vegetarians.

SATURATED FATS contain no unsaturated bonds. High intakes raise blood cholesterol levels and blood fat levels. Saturated fats are mainly found in full-cream dairy products, meat, coconut and palm oil.

TRANS-FATTY ACIDS are formed during the hydrogenation process that turns oils into solid fats. The body cannot use trans-fatty acids and they have been shown to increase 'bad' cholesterol levels and decrease 'good' cholesterol levels. Fats high in trans-fatty acids are mainly used to manufacture biscuits, pastries and cakes, and for frying in some fast-food restaurants. Polyunsaturated and monounsaturated margarines now contain minimal levels, and some are trans-fatty-acid free. Trans-fatty acids also occur naturally in meat, milk and cheese.

VITAMINS are complex chemicals found in food and needed by the body in minute quantities. They are essential for growth, development, metabolism and health.

FOOD LABELLING

Throughout this book, we recommend that you read food labels carefully to determine the amount of fat, fibre and carbohydrate in packaged foods. But what does all that information on the packet mean?

MEASURE This tells you the weight of the food without the packaging.

NAME OF FOOD Certain foods are required by law to be sold under prescribed names, such as margarine, ice cream and bread, and contain specified quantities of ingredients.

NUTRITION INFORMATION PANEL This panel must be provided by the manufacturer if they make a nutritional claim anywhere on their packaging. The panel lists nutritional information per serving and per 100 g (which allows you to compare different products).

NAME AND ADDRESS The manufacturer, packer or importer is required to state a contact name and address.

INGREDIENTS Manufacturers must list the ingredients in order of decreasing weight (except for water). The number of any additive is listed next to its function, such as preservative or colour.

COUNTRY OF ORIGIN A confusing label as it can mean the country in which the food was grown or the country in which it was packaged.

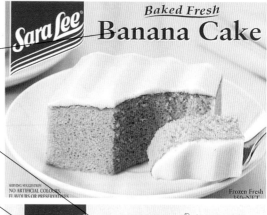

Baked Fresh

Banana Cake

350gNET

Baked Fresh
Banana Cake

SERVING SUGGESTION
NO ARTIFICIAL COLOURS,
FLAVOURS OR PRESERVATIVES

Frozen Fresh
350gNET

NUTRITION INFORMATION		
SERVINGS PER PACK 6	PER	PER
SERVING SIZE: 58g	SERVE	100g
ENERGY	856kJ	1475kJ
PROTEIN	1.7g	3.0g
FAT	7.2g	12.4g
CARBOHYDRATE		
-TOTAL	32.9g	56.7g
-SUGARS	21.6g	37.3g
SODIUM	219mg	378mg
POTASSIUM	82mg	142mg

Sara Lee outer packaging and foil is fully recyclable.

9 310135 026617

WE VALUE YOUR OPINION. FOR COMMENTS OR FURTHER INFORMATION ABOUT SARA LEE PRODUCTS PHONE FREECALL 1800 065 056 PLEASE RETAIN ALL PACKAGING

SARA LEE BAKERY (AUSTRALIA) PTY LTD
RAILWAY CRESCENT, LISAROW, GOSFORD 2250
INGREDIENTS: BANANA [FOOD ACID (330)], SUGAR, FLOUR, FRESH EGG, FONDANT [SUCROSE, GLUCOSE, WATER ADDED], VEGETABLE FATS AND OILS, BUTTER, EMULSIFIER (471), GLUCOSE, BAKING POWDER, THICKENER (1412), SALT, BAKING SODA, VANILLA (NATURAL), VEGETABLE GUM (414), WATER ADDED.
STORE AT OR BELOW -18°C.
NO ARTIFICIAL COLOURS, FLAVOURS OR PRESERVATIVES.
MADE IN AUSTRALIA.

DID YOU KNOW?

LIGHT This doesn't mean low in fat, it means light in colour, weight or texture. This is significant when buying oils, as all oils, light or regular, have the same fat content.

REDUCED FAT To be labelled reduced fat, sugar, salt or energy, a food must be reduced by at least 25% compared to the regular product. This doesn't mean it's low in fat, just lower in fat than the original—reduced-fat milk has 2% fat, but reduced-fat cheese has 25% fat.

CHOLESTEROL FREE Not the same as fat-free. Many 'cholesterol-free' foods in fact have plenty of fat. To lower cholesterol, concentrate instead on cutting out saturated fat.

HOW TO USE THIS BOOK

On the left-hand pages are tables that list the carbohydrate, fibre, fat and energy content of foods. The right-hand pages give information, ideas and tips about food and health. Use the tables and text together to plan and manage a healthy diet— the tables provide the facts, while the text provides the inspiration.

The figure next to each food in the tables represents the average serving size. This is the best way of seeing how much fat, fibre and carbohydrate you are really getting in a bowl of cereal or a slice of bread.

For foods like flour that don't have a serving size, we have used a 100 g amount, which is the easiest way to compare similar products. When N/T appears in a column, it means that the food has not been tested

nutritionally in this category.

The text on the right-hand page focuses on one food from the opposite table, and gives you the information you need to achieve a balanced diet. It contains tips on how to switch high-fat foods for low-fat ones without even noticing; delicious, easy recipes; essential information on the best choices for everyday shopping; and even advises which foods help protect against illness.

A HEALTHY MENU FOR A DAY

BREAKFAST

Start with an orange, grapefruit, melon or paw paw (all high in Vitamin C).
Then choose from:

A bowl of wholegrain cereal or untoasted muesli and 2 slices of wholegrain toast
OR
Baked beans on toast
OR
1 bowl of porridge (use fruit instead of sugar to sweeten)
OR
A banana smoothie made with low-fat milk and honey.

MID-MEAL SNACKS

Keep your energy levels high with a low-fat yoghurt, dried fruit or a fresh fruit salad.

LUNCH

Accompany your lunch with a couple of glasses of water.

A lentil burger on wholegrain bread
OR
Californian rolls with miso soup
OR
A bowl of chunky vegetable soup with a bagel
OR
Niçoise salad with oil-free dressing
OR
Baked potato with salmon, capers and low-fat yoghurt
OR
Roll-up with hummus, tabouli and skin-free chicken

Finish with a piece of fruit.

DINNER

Don't make this the big meal of the day—spread out your eating more evenly.

Barbecued fillet steak with spicy chutney and chargrilled vegetables
OR
Chilli con carne with rice
OR
Mushroom risotto
OR
Chargrilled tuna or salmon with salsa, steamed potatoes and vegetables
OR
Spicy vegetables with steamed couscous

Finish with poached fruit, a baked apple or a grilled banana with low-fat yoghurt.

FOOD	CARB	FIBRE	FAT	ENERGY
	g	g	g	kJ
AGAR				
dried, 100 g	81	8	0.5	1280
soaked, 100 g	7	0.5	0	110
ALCOHOL				
ale, average, 375 ml	5	0	0	535
beer, average, 375 ml	7.5	0	0	560
beer, Castlemaine XXXX, 375 ml	7	0	0	550
beer, Castlemaine XXXX Light Bitter, 375 ml	3	0	0	440
beer, Fosters Lager; Victoria Bitter, 375 ml	7.5	0	0	600
beer, Tooheys Red, 375 ml	7.5	0	0	660
beer, reduced-alcohol, Coopers Light, 375 ml	7.5	0	0	360
beer, reduced-alcohol, Fosters Lite Ice, 375 ml	7.5	0	0	395
champagne, average, 120 ml	1	0	0	325
cider, draught, Strongbow, 375 ml	11	0	0	695
cider, dry, Strongbow, 375 ml	11	0	0	585
cider, sweet, Strongbow, 375 ml	25	0	0	820
cider, white, Strongbow, 375 ml	26	0	0	890
cocktail, Bloody Mary, 165 ml	5.5	0.5	0	520
cocktail, Daiquiri, 60 ml	4	0	0	465
cocktail, Tequila Sunrise, 60 ml	7	0	0	275
liqueur, Advocaat, 30 ml	8.5	0	0	340
liqueur, Benedictine; Galliano; Sambuca, 30 ml	N/T	0	0	440
liqueur, cherry brandy, 30 ml	10	0	0	325
liqueur, Curacao, 30 ml	8.5	0	0	390
liqueur, Grand Marnier, 30 ml	N/T	0	0	420
liqueur, Kirsch, 30 ml	N/T	0	0	355
liqueur, Baileys; Drambuie; Malibu, 30 ml	N/T	0	0	420
spirits, average, 30 ml	0	0	0	270
spirits, Bacardi, 30 ml	0	0	0	275
spirits, brandy, 30 ml	0	0	0	270
spirits, gin, 30 ml	0	0	0	260
spirits, rum, 30 ml	0	0	0	265
spirits, vodka, 30 ml	0	0	0	265
spirits, whisky, 30 ml	0	0	0	270
stout, Coopers, 375 ml	14	0	0	810
stout, Guinness, 375 ml	18	0	0	940
wine, red, dry; rosé, 120 ml	2.5	0	0	335
wine, red, sweet, 120 ml	2	0	0	355
wine, rice, sake, 100 ml	N/T	0	0	460
wine, Sauternes, 120 ml	0	0	0	560
wine, white, dry, 120 ml	0.5	0	0	340
wine, white, sweet, 120 ml	3	0	0	330
wine, fortified, port, 60 ml	7.5	0	0	360
wine, fortified, sherry, dry, 60 ml	1	0	0	260
wine, fortified, sherry, sweet, 60 ml	6.5	0	0	345
wine, fortified, vermouth, dry, 60 ml	2	0	0	270
wine, fortified, vermouth, sweet, 60 ml	9	0	0	355

ALCOHOL The debate continues about whether alcohol should be incorporated as a healthy part of our daily diet. A couple of glasses each day is thought to decrease the risk of heart disease, but it can still be a good idea to have an alcohol-free day each week. Eat before drinking to lessen the temptation to snack on high-fat chips and peanuts.

BEER A concentrated form of kilojoules, beer and other drinks also weaken your resolve. Many people reach for high-fat snacks after a few drinks.

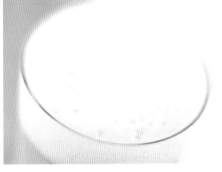

RECIPE For a refreshing summer drink with just 165 kilojoules, pour equal amounts of champagne and soda over berries or peaches and stand for a few minutes before drinking.

WHITE WINE Mix with ice-cold soda to make a wine spritzer with half the kilojoules of a glass of wine.

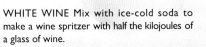

SPIRITS Mixing an alcoholic drink with coke or juice increases the kilojoules.

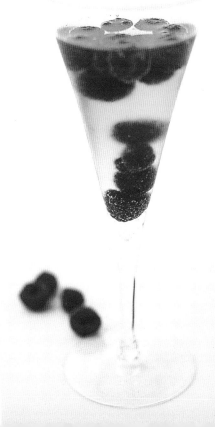

FOOD	CARB g	FIBRE g	FAT g	ENERGY kJ
APPLE				
canned pieces, no sugar, 1 cup, 220 g	20	2	0	335
cider, non-alcoholic, 1 glass, 250 ml	25	0	0	415
dried, 30 g	25	5	0	395
juice, no sugar, 1 glass, 250 ml	26.5	0	0	420
juice drink (frozen concentrate), diluted, 1 cup, 250 ml	29	0	0	490
raw, peeled, 1 medium, 100 g	12	1	0	205
raw, unpeeled, 1 medium, 120 g	15	2.5	0	250
snack pack, 1 cup, 135 g	30	5	1	440
stuffed & baked, 1 medium, 250 g	33.5	4	0.5	580
APRICOT				
canned in juice, drained, 6 halves	9	2	0	170
canned in syrup, drained, 6 halves	12	2	0	210
canned in water, no sugar, 6 halves	4.5	1.5	0	95
dried, 3 whole, 50 g	22	4.5	0	410
juice drink, 35% juice, 1 glass, 250 ml	20	1	0	75
nectar, 50% juice, 1 glass, 250 ml	32	0	0	540
raw, 1 medium, 56 g	4	1	0	85
ARROWROOT 1 tbsp	8.5	0	0	145
ARTICHOKE				
globe, boiled, 1 medium, 120 g	1.5	1	0	105
hearts, canned in brine, drained, 1 heart, 50 g	1	1.5	0	35
Jerusalem, peeled, boiled, 1 medium, 100 g	3	3	0	105
ASPARAGUS				
canned, drained, 8 spears	2	4.5	0	85
fresh, boiled, 2 spears, 50 g	1	1	0	40
AVOCADO all varieties, 1/2 medium, 95 g	0.5	2	25	1055
BABY FOOD				
baby rusk, teething, Heinz, 100 g	58.5	4.5	2	1350
baby rusk, teething, Vegetable, Heinz, 100 g	9.1	4.5	3	1550
baby rusk, toddler teething, Cheddar Cheese, Heinz, 100 g	71	4.5	8.5	1765
cereal, ground muesli, 100 g	70	7	8	1690
cereal, High-protein Cereal, Heinz, 100 g	58	6	5.5	1510
cereal, Muesli & Fruit, Heinz, 100 g	71	7	8	1690
cereal, Original Blended, Farex, 100 g	75.5	3	2	1565
cereal, Rice, Farex, 100 g	78	2	4	1580
cereal, Rice, Heinz, 100 g	78	2	4	1580
dessert, Apple & Apricot Muesli, Only Organic, 1 jar, 128 g	8	N/T	0.5	155
dessert, Apricots & Rice, Heinz, 100 g	16.5	N/T	0	300
dessert, Banana Rice Pudding, Only Organic, 1 jar, 128 g	10.5	N/T	1.5	270
dessert, Caramel Custard, Heinz, 100 g	13	N/T	2.5	345
dessert, Fruit Custard, Heinz, 100 g	17	N/T	0.5	310
dinner, Beef, Heinz Junior, 100 g	10	1	0.5	240
dinner, Chicken, Heinz Junior, 100 g	9	0.5	1	230

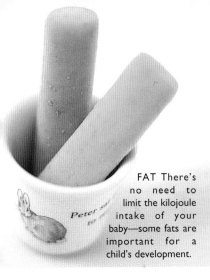

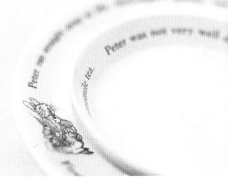

BEST FOR BABY For the first 6 months, breast milk or formula, rather than solid food, is a baby's major source of nutrition and provides all the vitamins, minerals and kilojoules a baby needs.

FAT There's no need to limit the kilojoule intake of your baby—some fats are important for a child's development.

BABY FOOD Keep it simple and nutritious, with lots of puréed fruits and vegetables. Commercial baby foods are prepared under strict conditions and can be a convenient way to feed your baby. Babies don't need extra salt or sugar, so check food labels, but don't give babies and young children reduced-fat or skim milk as they lack vitamins and kilojoules.

FIBRE You can start introducing more solid food, including high-fibre wholemeal bread and cereals, when the baby is over 6 months.

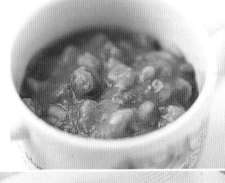

RECIPE To make a nutritious meal for your baby, high in carbohydrates and fibre, steam some pumpkin and potato until tender. Purée with a little cold water, then pass through a sieve to remove any lumps.

FOOD	CARB	FIBRE	FAT	ENERGY
	g	g	g	kJ
dinner, Chicken Noodle, Heinz Junior, 100 g	9.5	0.5	1	240
dinner, Chicken & Vegetable, Heinz, 100 g	8	1.5	1.5	250
dinner, Garden Vegetable, Only Organic, 200 g	24	N/T	0.5	520
dinner, Lamb, Heinz Junior, 100 g	7	1	2.5	260
dinner, Lamb Casserole, Only Organic, 1 jar, 200 g	18	N/T	2	510
dinner, Lentil Hot-pot, Only Organic, 1 jar, 200 g	20	N/T	0.5	480
dinner, Mixed Vegetable, strained, Heinz, 100 g	8.5	N/T	1	195
dinner, Wholemeal Pasta & Vegetable, Only Organic, 1 jar, 200 g	27	N/T	1	580
BACON				
bits, 2 teaspoons	0	0	1.5	125
fried & 2 fried eggs	0	0	18	905
lean, grilled & 2 poached eggs	0	0	9	540
middle rasher, fried, 1, 10 g	0	0	3	155
middle rasher, trimmed, fried, 1, 10 g	0	0	1	95
middle rasher, grilled, 1, 10 g	0	0	2	135
middle rasher, trimmed, grilled, 1, 10 g	0	0	1	100
BAGEL plain, Sara Lee, 1, 60 g	29	1.5	0.5	575
BAKLAVA commercial, average piece, 100 g	42	2	19.5	1540
BAMBOO SHOOTS				
canned or bottled, drained, 1 cup, 140 g	1.5	3	0	45
raw, 50 g	3	0	0	60
BANANA				
chips, 20 chips, 22 g	13	1.5	7.5	480
dried, 100 g	28	3	0	500
raw, peeled, 1, 140 g	28	3	1	500
smoothie, 1 glass, 300 ml	49.5	3	15.5	1585
sugar, raw, peeled, 1, 60 g	15	2	0	270
BARLEY				
bran, raw, 40 g	30	5	1	550
cooked, 1 cup, 180 g	38	6.5	1.5	800
pearl, cooked, 100 g	21	3.5	1	445
quick-cook, cooked, 100 g	70	13	3	1275
BEANS				
adzuki, cooked, 100 g	25	18.5	0	535
baked, canned, 100 g	11	5	0.5	285
black, cooked, salted, 100 g	23.5	8.5	0.5	550
black-eyed, cooked, 100 g	21	6.5	0.5	485
black gram, cooked, 100 g	13.5	6	0.5	380
black kidney (turtle), cooked, 100 g	24.5	5.5	0.5	545
borlotti, canned, drained, 100 g	25	6.5	0.5	470
borlotti, cooked, 100 g	28.5	11.5	0.5	612
broad, fresh, cooked, 100 g	2	4	0.5	175
butter (cannellini), fresh, cooked, 100 g	2	3	0	80
green, fresh, 100 g	2.5	2.5	0	85
green, frozen, cooked, 100 g	3	3	0	80

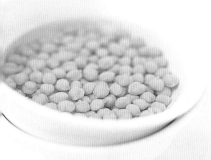

KIDNEY BEANS Next time you make chilli con carne, try using more kidney beans and less beef mince, as kidney beans are high in fibre and supply all the protein of meat without the fat.

CHICKPEAS Readily available in tins, chickpeas are a great source of fibre and a cheap, low-fat alternative to meat.

BEANS
Rich in protein, dietary fibre and complex carbohydrates, and low in fat, beans should be an essential part of our diet, especially for people who don't eat any or much meat. The canned varieties are great if you don't have time to soak dried beans overnight.

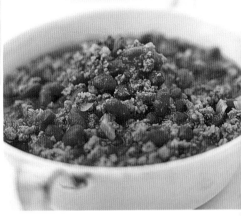

SOYA BEANS Much talked about by nutritionists, soya beans are an excellent source of phytoestrogens, which can benefit menopausal women. Soya beans also provide the best-quality protein of all the pulses.

RECIPE Process chickpeas with a little tahini, garlic, lemon juice, oil and water to make a delicious low-fat dip. Serve with pieces of wholemeal lavash or Lebanese bread that have been baked until crisp.

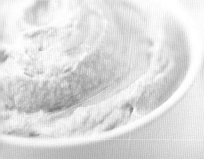

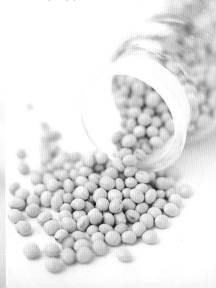

FOOD	CARB	FIBRE	FAT	ENERGY
	g	g	g	kJ
haricot, cooked, 100 g	12.5	9	0.5	375
kidney, red, canned, drained, cooked, 100 g	13	6.5	0.5	360
kidney, red, dried, 100 g	9	7	0.5	310
lima, canned, drained, 100 g	15	5	0.5	330
lima, dried, cooked, 100 g	10	5.5	0.5	295
Mexe, Old El Paso, 100 g	14.5	5.5	0.5	350
mung, cooked, 100 g	19	7.5	0.5	440
pinto, cooked, 100 g	25.5	8.5	0.5	575
purple, cooked, 100 g	2.5	4.5	0.5	120
runner, cooked, 100 g	0	2.5	0	85
Refried, Old El Paso, 100 g	13.5	4.5	1	340
Refried with Green Chillies, Old El Paso, 100 g	13.5	4.5	1	340
snake, cooked, 100 g	2	4	0	95
soya, canned, drained, 100 g	2	5	5.5	385
soya, canned in tomato sauce, 100 g	7	3	3	380
soya, dried, cooked, 100 g	1.5	7	7.5	540
three-bean mix, canned, drained, 100 g	14	6	0.5	360
BEEF				
blade steak, lean, grilled, 1, 117 g	0	0	10.5	940
blade steak, untrimmed, grilled, 1, 120 g	0	0	12.5	1040
chuck steak, untrimmed, simmered, 1, 190 g	0	0	26	2040
corned, canned, 100 g	0.5	0	11	805
corned, lean, 100 g	0	0	2.5	410
corned, untrimmed, 100 g	0	0	9	625
corned & cereal, canned, 100 g	5	1.5	13.5	825
corned silverside (sandwich), 75% trim, 60 g	0	0	3.5	380
fillet steak, lean, grilled, 1 small, 85 g	0	0	7	700
fillet steak, untrimmed, grilled, 1 small, 85 g	0	0	11	830
hamburger patties, Big Beefers, I & J, 1 patty, 100 g	0.5	0	20	1054
hamburger patties, Lean Beefers, I & J, 1 patty, 100 g	0.5	0	7	555
heart, simmered, 100 g	0	0	2.5	625
kidney, simmered, 100 g	0	0	2.5	565
liver, simmered, 100 g	0	0	11.5	925
mince, hamburger, simmered, drained, 170 g	0	0	20.5	1530
mince, regular, simmered, drained, 170 g	0	0	16.5	1300
oxtail, simmered, 100 g	0	0	29.5	1450
pepper steak with cream sauce, 1 serve, 200 g	0	0	35	2250
pie, commercial, family size, 1 serve, 250 g	38.5	3	36.5	2355
pie, commercial, individual, 250 g	45	3	34.5	2370
pie, commercial, party, 1, 40 g	7.5	0.5	7.5	465
rib eye steak, lean, grilled, 1 small steak, 110 g	0	0	9	910
rib eye steak, untrimmed, grilled, 1 small steak, 130 g	0	0	20.5	1390
rib steak (porterhouse), lean, grilled, 100 g	0	0	5.5	740
rissoles, fried, 2, 340 g	0	3.5	30	2780
round steak, lean, grilled, 100 g	0	0	6	740

CASEROLES To make your casseroles lower in kilojoules but still full of flavour, prepare one day in advance and refrigerate overnight. Before reheating, carefully lift off and discard the fat that will have risen and set on the surface.

MINCE To make really lean mince, buy lean steak and mince it yourself in a food processor. Alternatively, buy lean mince, which has half the fat of hamburger mince.

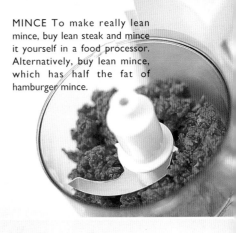

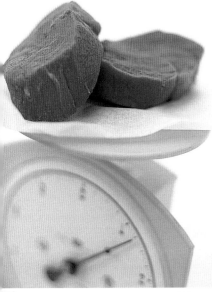

BEEF An excellent source of protein that doesn't have to be high in fat. Look for lean cuts that have had all visible fat removed and don't have much marbling, though do remember that fat tenderises the beef and lean cuts can be dry if overcooked. For a high-flavour, low-fat marinade, try any combination of lemon juice, mustard, soy sauce, wine or herbs.

RECIPE To give a fillet steak extra flavour when you are grilling or frying it without fat, baste with a little marinade of soy sauce, spread both sides with wholegrain mustard or coat in cracked black pepper.

COOKING To avoid adding extra fat, cook your meat on a lightly oiled griddle pan or barbecue, but don't turn the meat too often and allow to rest before serving to keep it from drying out.

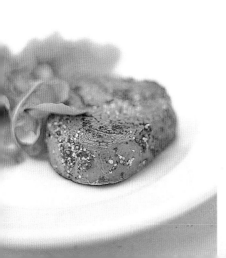

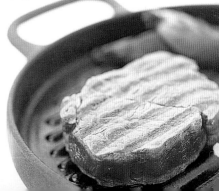

FOOD	CARB	FIBRE	FAT	ENERGY
	g	g	g	kJ
round steak, untrimmed, grilled, 100 g	0	0	9.5	850
rump steak, lean, grilled, 1, 175 g	0	0	11.5	1405
rump steak, untrimmed, grilled, 1, 200 g	0	0	33.5	2260
silverside, lean, baked, 2 slices, 80 g	0	0	3.5	550
silverside, untrimmed, baked, 2 slices, 85 g	0	0	10	795
sirloin steak, lean, grilled, 1, 110 g	0	0	9.5	890
sirloin steak, untrimmed, grilled, 1, 127 g	0	0	24	1460
skirt steak, lean, simmered, 100 g	0	0	5	790
skirt steak, untrimmed, simmered, 100 g	0	0	6	825
T-bone, lean, grilled, 100 g	0	0	5.5	565
T-bone, untrimmed, grilled, 100 g	0	0	8	690
tongue, simmered, 100 g	0	0	25	1290
topside roast, lean, baked, 2 slices, 80 g	0	0	4	520
topside roast, untrimmed, baked, 2 slices, 90 g	0	0	9	720
topside steak, lean, grilled, 1 small steak, 100 g	0	0	5	635
topside steak, untrimmed, grilled, 1 small steak, 100 g	0	0	6.5	680
tournedos, grilled, 1 medium fillet	0	1	20	1780
tripe, simmered, 100 g	0	0	3	350
BEETROOT				
canned, 5 slices, 100 g	14	4	0	270
fresh, peeled, boiled, 2 slices	5	1.5	0	105
raw, grated, 30 g	2.5	1	0	50
BELGIAN ENDIVE (WITLOF) raw, 1 head, 60 g	0	1.5	0	25
BISCUITS (SEE ALSO CRISPBREAD)				
Adora Creams, Arnotts, 1	4	0	1.5	120
Assorted Creams, Westons, 1	12.5	0	4	315
Aussie Macadamia, Westons, 1	8	0	4	300
Blackforest Cherry, Westons, 1	10	0	3.5	360
chocolate, Butternut Snaps, Arnotts, 1	11.5	0.5	4	370
chocolate, Caramel Crowns, Arnotts, 1	10.5	0.5	4	345
chocolate, Chocolate Chip, Farmbake, Arnotts, 1	4.5	0	2	150
chocolate, Fruit & Nut, Arnotts, 1	8.5	0.5	3.5	275
chocolate, Gaiety, Arnotts, 1	8	0	4	300
chocolate, Granita, Arnotts, 1	10.5	0.5	4	355
chocolate, Jamaican, Westons, 1	11.5	0	4	355
chocolate, Mint Slices, Arnotts, 1	5.5	0	4	345
chocolate, Monte, Arnotts, 1	8	0	3.5	280
chocolate, Royals, dark, Arnotts, 1	10.5	0	3.5	310
chocolate, Royals, milk, Arnotts, 1	10.5	0	3	315
chocolate, Scotch Finger, Arnotts, 1	14.5	0.5	5.5	490
chocolate, Tim Tams, Arnotts, 1	11.5	0	5	400
chocolate, Tiny Teddy, Arnotts, 1	1.5	0	0.5	35
cookies, Anzac, Westons, 1	9	0	2.5	260
cookies, Butternut, Arnotts, 1	8.5	0.5	2.5	255
cookies, Cornflake, Westons, 1	8.5	N/T	3	270
cookies, Wizard, Westons, 1	9	0	3	270

BISCUITS

Sweet biscuits are often high in sugar and saturated fat, but they can be useful as a quick source of carbohydrate. If you want something more low fat to snack on, reach for fresh or dried fruit, or a crispbread or rice cake with cottage cheese or peanut butter. Alternatively, baking your own biscuits will let you cut back on fat and sugar.

SHORTBREAD

High in fat and sugar, that lovely melt-in-the-mouth texture comes from the high ratio of butter to flour.

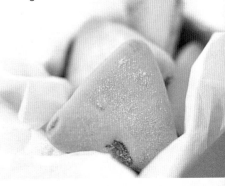

COOKIES

Chewy ones get their texture from the high amount of butter and sugar. Don't be fooled into thinking oatmeal biscuits are lower in fat, though they do contain more fibre.

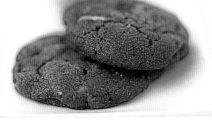

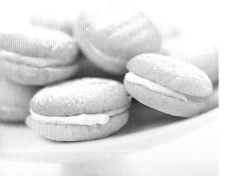

BISCOTTI

A great low-fat biscuit. Made with eggs, they contain no butter and because they contain nuts, they also have extra fibre.

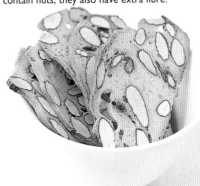

CREAM-FILLED

High in fat and sugar, the centre is usually a mix of icing sugar, butter and water, and in most cases the biscuit is sweet and buttery.

LOW-FAT

There are biscuits now available in supermarkets that are up to 70% lower in fat than normal biscuits. Fruit juice is often used to sweeten the mixture instead of sugar.

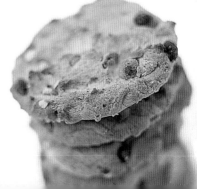

FOOD	CARB	FIBRE	FAT	ENERGY
	g	g	g	kJ
cookies, Lots O' Chips, Westons, 1	8.5	0	3	270
Coconut Ice, Westons, 1	9.5	0	3.5	300
Cool Dudes, Westons, 1	7.5	0	2.5	225
Delta Creams, Arnotts, 1	10	0	3.5	310
Full 'O' Fruit, Arnotts, 1	7.5	0.5	0.5	160
Ginger Nuts, Arnotts, 1	10.5	0.5	1.5	240
Golliwog, Arnotts, 1	8	0.5	1.5	200
Granita, Arnotts, 1	8	0.5	2.5	245
Honey Snaps, Arnotts, 1	4.5	0	1	120
Iced Vo-Vos, Arnotts, 1	9.5	0.5	1.5	230
Italian Cappuccino, Westons, 1	9.5	0	3	280
Jamaican Ginger, Westons, 1	8.5	0	2.5	240
Milk Coffee, Arnotts, 1	7	0	1	160
Milk Coffee, Westons, 1	6.5	0	1.5	170
Morning Coffee, Arnotts, 1	4.5	0	1	115
Morning Coffee, Westons, 1	6	0	1	125
Nice, Arnotts, 1	9	0.5	2	235
Pebbles, Westons, 1	9.5	0	7.5	270
savoury, BBQ Shapes, Arnotts, 1	1.5	0	0.5	55
savoury, Breton, Arnotts, 1	2.5	0.5	1	90
savoury, Breton, reduced-salt, Arnotts, 1	2.5	0.5	1	90
savoury, Cheddar Shapes, Arnotts, 1	2.5	0	0.5	75
savoury, Chicken Crimpy Shapes, Arnotts, 1	2	0	0.5	60
savoury, Cracked Pepper Shapes, Arnotts, 1	3	0	1	85
savoury, Savoury Shapes, Arnotts, 1	1	0	0.5	35
shortbread, Amo, Arnotts, 1	7.5	0.5	3	255
shortbread, Cream, Arnotts, 1	10.5	0	4.5	365
shortbread, Scotch Finger, Arnotts, 1	12	0.5	4	370
Snack Right, Choc-chip, Arnotts, 1	8	0	2	215
Snack Right, Fruit Slice, Arnotts, 1	8	0.5	0.5	155
Snack Right, Golden Oat, Arnotts, 1	9.5	0.5	1.5	225
Snack Right, Kingston, Arnotts, 1	9.5	0.5	2.5	270
Snack Right, Monte Carlo, Arnotts, 1	16	0.5	3	400
Teddy Playtime, Westons, 1	5.5	0	1.5	155
Venetian, Arnotts, 1	8	0	3.5	280
BITTER MELON (BALSAM PEAR) raw, 1, 100 g	0	2	0	20
BLACKBERRIES				
canned, sweetened, 100 g	23	3.5	0	385
fresh, raw, 1/2 punnet, 100 g	12.5	5.5	0.5	220
frozen, 100 g	15.5	5	0.5	270
BLACKCURRANT JUICE prepared, Ribena, Smithkline Beecham, 250 ml	28	0	0	450
BLUEBERRIES				
canned in syrup, drained, 100 g	17	4	0	290
frozen, 100 g	12	2.5	0.5	215
raw, 1/2 punnet, 100 g	14	2.5	0.5	235
BOYSENBERRIES				
canned in heavy syrup, 100 g	22.5	2.5	0	370

FLAVOURED CRACKERS These tend to be high in fat, salt and artificial flavours. Crackers that are baked instead of fried may still have a lot of fat.

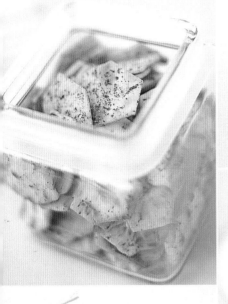

BISCUITS, CRACKERS & CRISPBREADS Savoury biscuits can be low in fat and sugar and provide a tasty alternative to bread for sandwiches. Those with added cereal grains often have high levels of dietary fibre, making them a great choice for a nutritious energy boost. Read the labels though, as some varieties are high in fat.

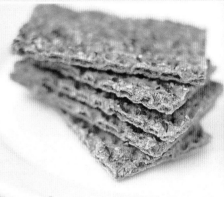

WATER CRACKERS Relatively fat-free, these crackers are a good source of carbohydrate. Dip into a low-fat dip made from low-fat yoghurt mixed with sweet chilli sauce or coriander, or refried beans with a little tomato salsa.

CRISPBREADS A high-fibre choice for an afternoon snack. Top with some cottage or low-fat soft cheese and slices of ripe tomato.

RICE CRACKERS A tasty low-fat cracker that provides a handy gluten-free snack high in carbohydrate.

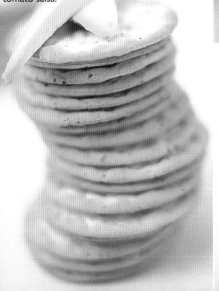

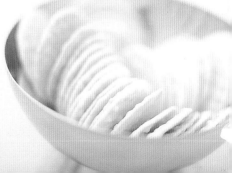

FOOD	CARB	FIBRE	FAT	ENERGY
	g	g	g	kJ
canned, no added sugar, 100 g	4	4	0	115
raw, 1/2 punnet, 100 g	6	5	0	155
BRAN (SEE CEREAL)				
BRANDY BUTTER 1 1/2 tbsps, 30 g	16	0	8	615
BRAWN 2 slices, 70 g	0	0	12	635
BREAD				
bagel, plain, Sara Lee, 1, 60 g	29	1.5	0.5	575
corn, 90 g	20	2.5	7	750
crumpet, regular, toasted, 1, 45 g	19.5	1	0.5	390
crumpet, wholemeal, toasted, 1, 44 g	17	1.5	0.5	355
damper, commercial, 1 thick slice, 60 g	35	1	6	810
flat, chapati, 1, 100 g	35	3	1.5	780
flat, focaccia, 1, 50 g	30	2	1.5	585
flat, Focaccia, Herb & Garlic, Tip Top, 1, 70 g	32	2	1.5	715
flat, Lavash, Tip Top, 1, 60 g	35	2.5	1.5	750
flat, Lavash, yeast-free, 1, 60 g	35	2.5	1.5	750
flat, Lebanese, white, 1, 110 g	57	3	2.5	1230
flat, Lebanese, wholemeal, 1, 110 g	50	7	2	1090
flat, naan, 1, 60 g	310	1.5	8	850
flat, pita, 1 large, 60 g	35	2.5	1	670
flat, pita, Egyptian, white, 1, 35 g	18	1	0.5	380
flat, pita, Egyptian, wholemeal, 1, 35 g	17	1	2	375
flat, tortilla, wheat flour, 1, 30 g	15	1	2	360
flat, Turkish, 1, 50 g	N/T	N/T	0.5	535
garlic, commercial, 2 slices, 65 g	35	1.5	11.5	1140
loaf, Energy Plus, Uncle Tobys, 2 slices	35	3.5	2	795
loaf, fruit, Fruit & Spice, Buttercup, 2 slices	34.5	3.5	2	745
loaf, fruit, Raisin Toast, Tip Top, 2 slices	26	2	1.5	565
loaf, fruit, Spicy Fruit, Tip Top, 2 slices	33.5	2.5	2	730
loaf, gluten/wheat/yeast-free, Moores, 2 slices	12	2	2	270
loaf, Grains Plus, Uncle Tobys, 2 slices	35	5	2	785
loaf, mixed grain, Fruit Loaf, Burgen, 2 slices	33.5	3.5	3.5	825
loaf, multigrain, 9 Grain, Tip Top, 2 slices	26	5	3	695
loaf, multigrain, Tip Top, 2 slices	26.5	3	1.5	610
loaf, Oat Bran & Honey, Burgen, 2 slices	28	5	4	810
loaf, pumpernickel, 2 slices	18	5	1	385
loaf, Rice Bran, Moores, 2 slices	2	1	10	290
loaf, Black Rye, Riga, 1 slice	42	7	2	900
loaf, Rye, Burgen, 2 slices	30	4.5	3	740
loaf, Soy & Linseed, Burgen, 2 slices	40	6.5	6	1090
loaf, Soy & Linseed, Molenberg, Buttercup, 2 slices	30.5	N/T	4.5	855
loaf, Soy & Linseed, Vogel, 2 slices	26	8	5	790
loaf, Sunflower & Barley, Riga, 2 slices	35	5	2.5	815
loaf, Vita Gold, Uncle Tobys, 2 slices	35	5.5	1.5	780
loaf, white, Hyfibe, Tip Top, 2 slices	29	4	2	675
loaf, white, Sunblest Toast, Tip Top, 2 slices	31.5	4	2	725
loaf, white, Super Sandwich Maker, Buttercup, 2 slices	30	2	1.5	655

WHITE A good source of protein, fibre, vitamins and minerals, even if it is not quite as nutritious as wholemeal bread. White bread is low in fat.

WHOLEMEAL AND MIXED GRAIN Both have more fibre and vitamins than white bread, with wholemeal having the most.

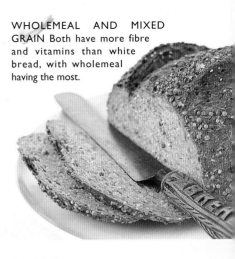

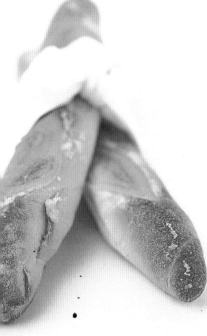

BREAD

Let's dispel the myth once and for all that bread is fattening—it is the spreads that we cover it with that can be. Bread provides us with dietary fibre, energy and valuable vitamins and minerals, and even white bread is nutritious. One pitfall is that commercial bread can be high in sodium—check the label for details.

HI-FIBRE A bread with added fibre, which gives it the same amount of fibre as wholemeal. Perfect for school packed lunches.

RYE Light rye has a similar nutritional value to white bread, whereas dark or black rye is a better source of fibre, iron and magnesium.

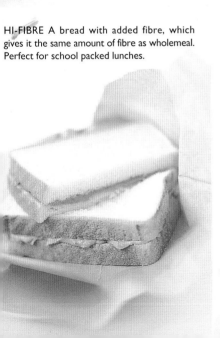

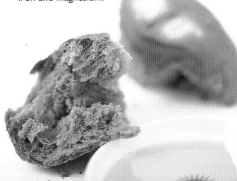

FOOD	CARB	FIBRE	FAT	ENERGY
	g	g	g	kJ
loaf, white, Super Toasty, Buttercup, 2 slices	35	2	1.5	755
loaf, white, Wonder White, Buttercup, 2 slices,	31.5	4	1.5	695
loaf, white, Wonder White Toast,				
Buttercup, 2 slices,	36.5	4.5	2	810
loaf, white/wholemeal, Light, Riga, 2 slices	18	2.5	1	405
loaf, wholemeal, Holsoms, Tip Top, 2 slices	31	4.5	2	705
loaf, wholemeal, Pritikin, Riga, 2 slices	28	3.5	1	595
loaf, Wholemeal & Sesame, Vogel, 2 slices	33	5.5	4.5	860
loaf, wholemeal, Tip Top, 2 slices	25.5	4	1.5	590
loaf, wholemeal, Traditional,				
Buttercup, 2 slices	28	4.5	1.5	635
roll, bap, 1, 60 g	31	2	2.5	680
roll, dinner, 1, 30 g	14.5	1	1	325
roll, Focaccia, Poppy Seed/Onion,				
Tip Top, 1, 70 g	32	2	1.5	715
roll, hamburger, 1, 60 g	29	2	1.5	650
roll, hotdog, 1, 43 g	21.5	1	2	515
roll, wholemeal, 1, 105 g	46	6	2.5	1050
stick, French (baguette), white, 1, 50 g	22.5	1.5	1.5	540
stick, French (baguette), wholemeal, 1, 50 g	21	2.5	1.5	500
stick, small, grissini, 1, 8 g	4	0	0.5	105
toast, French, 2 slices	20	1	8.5	765
BREADCRUMBS				
commercial, 1 cup, 180 g	59	4	3	1330
fresh, wholemeal, 1 cup, 180 g	70	12	5	1690
BREADFRUIT raw, 60 g	16	3	0	260
BROCCOLI raw, 100 g	0	4	0	100
BRUSSEL SPROUTS raw, 100 g	2	4	0	100
BUCKWHEAT KERNELS boiled, 100 g	73	5	2.5	1400
BULGUR (CRACKED WHEAT) cooked, 100 g	68.5	10.5	2.5	1340
BUN				
brioche, 1	N/T	N/T	16	1170
cinnamon, 1, 100 g	45	3	15	1105
cream, 1, 100 g	45	5	19	940
finger, iced, 1, 65 g	30	2	5	805
fruit, iced, 1, 90 g	42	3	7	1115
hot cross, 1, 40 g	20	1.5	1.5	455
BUTTER (SEE ALSO FAT AND MARGARINE)				
clarified (ghee), 1 tbsp	0	0	17	630
garlic, 1 tbsp	0	0	16.5	610
regular, average, 1 tbsp	0	0	16.5	610
reduced-fat, average, 1 tbsp	0	0	8	320
CABBAGE				
Chinese, raw, 1/2 cup, 40 g	0	1	0	14
Chinese, flowering (pak choi), raw, 40 g	0	1	0	20
mustard (dai gai choi), raw, 75 g	0.5	2	0	45
red, raw, 1/2 cup, 40 g	1	2	0	40
red, cooked, 1/2 cup, 60 g	2	2	0	50

BUTTER & MARGARINE Which

is healthier? In fact, they usually have the same fat content. Margarine is lower in saturated fat and cholesterol, but many people prefer butter as they feel it is a more natural product. As long as you don't eat too much, and your blood cholesterol level is not high, both butter and margarine are perfectly acceptable.

DAIRY SPREADS Gaining in popularity, these spreads have some canola or olive oil added, but they can still contain up to 42% saturated fat.

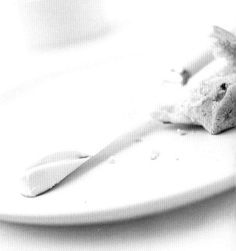

BUTTER By law, butter must contain over 80% fat. This fat is predominantly saturated and high in cholesterol.

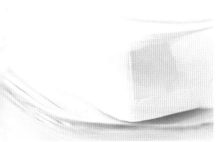

POLYUNSATURATED MARGARINES Made from sunflower, safflower and soya bean oils. You can lower blood cholesterol by replacing saturated fats with polyunsaturated fats. Some nuts and seeds contain polyunsaturated fats.

REDUCED-FAT SPREADS A blend of milk fat or vegetable oil and water, with about 50% of the fat of butter or margarine.

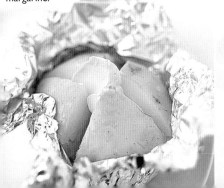

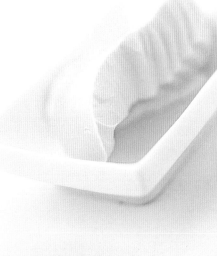

FOOD	CARB	FIBRE	FAT	ENERGY
	g	g	g	kJ
rolls, Lebanese, 3 small, 250 g	40	9	10	1220
Savoy, cooked, 1/2 cup, 60 g	1	2	0	40
Savoy, raw, 1/2 cup, 40 g	1	1	0	30
CAKE				
angel, average slice	40.5	0.5	0.5	760
Apricot Crumble Tea Cake, Sara Lee, 100 g	44	2	15	1360
apple, average slice	40	3	10	1060
Banana, Sara Lee, 100 g	57	2	12	1475
Banana Cake Fingers, Top Taste, 100 g	68	1.5	16	1800
Banana Madeira, Top Taste, 100 g	58	1.5	13.5	1540
Bavarian Chocolate, Sara Lee, 100 g	30	1	22.5	1395
Black Forest, Sara Lee, 100 g	40	1	17	1390
cake mix, Banana Cake, Greens, prepared, 1 slice, 50 g	27	N/T	8	1220
cake mix, Chocolate on Chocolate, White Wings, prepared, 1 slice, 90 g	49	N/T	8.5	1215
cake mix, Coconut & Banana, White Wings, prepared, 1 slice, 50 g	23.5	N/T	6	665
cake mix, Golden Butter Cake, Greens, prepared, 1 slice, 50 g	23	N/T	7	705
Cappuccino, Bon Gateaux, 75 g	N/T	N/T	17	1060
Cappuccino Rolls, Top Taste, 100 g	62	1	19	1840
Carrot, Sara Lee, 100 g	44	1	23	1690
Carrot Cake Fingers, Top Taste, 100 g	64	3	17	1770
Cheesecake Original, Sara Lee, 100 g	30	1	20	1350
Chocolate, Sara Lee, 100 g	55	1	17	1645
Christmas, 1 piece, 60 g	33.5	2	6	810
cup, iced, commercial, 1, 40 g	22.5	0.5	6	620
Date Loaf, White Wings, 1 piece, 55 g	27	3.5	4.5	665
date & walnut loaf, 1 piece, 60 g	32	3.5	6	795
eclair, chocolate, commercial, 70 g	22.5	0.5	18	1110
flan, fruit, 100 g	28.5	2	8	785
fruit, dark, commercial, 1 piece, 50 g	27	1.5	6	695
fruit, home-made, 1 piece, 70 g	39	2	7	945
Genoa, Top Taste, 100 g	59.5	N/T	12	1520
hazelnut torte, average slice	N/T	2.5	30	1690
Honey Rollettes, Top Taste, 100 g	63	N/T	11	1540
Jam Fairy, Top Taste, 100 g	58.5	N/T	18	1750
Jam Rollettes, Top Taste, 100 g	67.5	N/T	2.5	1310
lamington, commercial, 1, 75 g	36	1.5	9	980
Lamington, Cream-filled, Top Taste, 1, 60 g	30	2	7	785
Lemon Rollettes, Top Taste, 100 g	60.5	N/T	15	1510
Madeira, Top Taste, 100 g	52.5	N/T	14.5	1500
Madeira, Iced, Top Taste, 100 g	58	N/T	14	1550
Marble, Top Taste, 100 g	60	N/T	13.5	1570
Mud, Sara Lee, 100 g	59	1	20	1800
Napoleon, Top Taste, 100 g	59	N/T	18	1730
Passionfruit Squares, Top Taste, 100 g	65	N/T	13.5	1640

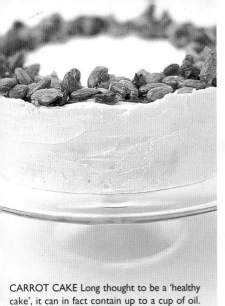

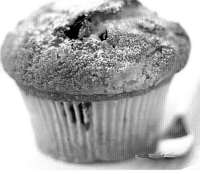

MUFFINS For healthy home-made muffins, use wholemeal self-raising flour to add fibre and replace the fat with half low-fat yoghurt and half orange juice.

CARROT CAKE Long thought to be a 'healthy cake', it can in fact contain up to a cup of oil. The cream cheese icing is high in fat and sugar.

ANGEL CAKE This cake is a weight-watcher's dream, as it contains no fat. It is made from egg whites and is high in sugar, but doesn't contain any butter or egg yolks.

CAKE As a general rule, the lighter and whiter the cake, the lower its fat content. Go for a sponge or angel cake rather than a rich yellow butter cake. Try making cakes with wholemeal flour to increase the fibre content, and use half whole eggs and half egg whites. Dried fruit cakes tend to be very moist and are made with less butter.

JAM ROLLETTES A jam filling is less fattening than a cream one, though jam will increase the sugar content.

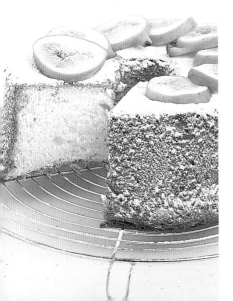

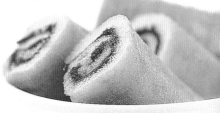

FOOD	CARB	FIBRE	FAT	ENERGY
	g	g	g	kJ
rock, 1 medium, 60 g	33	2	8	930
rum baba, average serve	47	1.5	10	1370
sponge, fairy, Top Taste, 100 g	60.5	N/T	8.5	1445
sponge, jam-filled, 1 slice, 30 g	16	0	2	380
Swiss roll, 1 slice, 35 g	22.5	0.5	2.5	480
CAPERS 1 tbsp	1	1	0	30
CAPSICUM				
green, raw, 100 g	2.5	1	0	65
red, raw, 100 g	4	1	0	105
CAROB				
bar, 1, 45 g	18	8	11.5	780
coated biscuit, 1, 18 g	9.5	0	5.5	375
powder, 2 tbsp, 40 g	15	0.5	0	250
CARROT				
baby, raw, peeled, 50 g	3	2	0	55
canned, 100 g	4	3	0	85
juice, 125 ml	8	5	0	165
raw, peeled, boiled, 1/2 cup, 70 g	4	2	0	80
CASSAVA peeled, boiled, 100 g	30.5	2	0.5	550
CAULIFLOWER				
boiled, 100 g	2	2	0	80
cheese, 200 g	11	2	20	1130
raw, 50 g	1	1	0	40
CELERIAC				
fresh, peeled, boiled, 100 g	5.5	5	0	130
fresh, peeled, 120 g	5	4.5	0	120
CELERY				
chopped, boiled, 1/2 cup, 63 g	1.5	1.5	0	35
raw, 2 × 10 cm sticks, 40 g	1	1	0.5	20
CEREAL				
4 Brans, 50 g	20	15	2	550
All-Bran, Kellogg's, 45 g	32.5	13	1.5	490
All-Bran Fruit'n Oats, Kellogg's, 45 g	34.5	9	1.5	580
bran, barley, Greens, 30 g	18	6	1	385
bran, natural, Purina, 12 g	7.5	4.5	0.5	140
bran, oat, unprocessed, 2 tbsp, 22 g	11	3.5	1.5	225
bran, rice, Greens, 15 g	7.5	4	3	295
bran, wheat, processed, 45 g	31	14	2.5	675
bran, wheat, unprocessed, 2 tbsp, 10 g	1	4.5	0.5	65
Bran Bix, Sanitarium, 40 g	21	9	1.5	505
Branflakes, Kellogg's, 30 g	23.5	4.5	0.5	470
Coco Pops, Kellogg's, 30 g	26	0.5	0	480
Cornflakes, Kellogg's, 30g	26	1	0	480
Cornflakes, Crunchy Nut, Kellogg's, 30 g	24.5	1.5	1	500
Cornpops, Kellogg's, 30 g	27	N/T	0	485
Crisppix, Kellogg's, 30 g	27	0.5	0	485
Crunchy Oat Bran with Fruit, Uncle Tobys, 45 g	31	6	2	675
Fibre Plus, Uncle Tobys, 45 g	29	7	1.5	620

CEREAL BRANS Dietary fibre can prevent cancer of the bowel and constipation, and cereal brans (the husks of grain) are a concentrated source. However, uncooked bran contains phytates that hinder the absorption of minerals. The best way to boost your fibre intake is with wholegrain cereals and breads, legumes, fruit and vegetables.

HIGH-FIBRE BREAKFAST Packed with fibre, baked beans on a piece of wholemeal toast or muffin is a great start to the day.

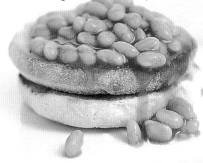

RECIPE Make a high-fibre smoothie by blending low-fat soya milk, yoghurt, a banana, honey and a tablespoon of oat bran.

BRAN CEREALS Processed bran cereals are a good high-fibre alternative to raw bran, but check the labels for added salt and sugar.

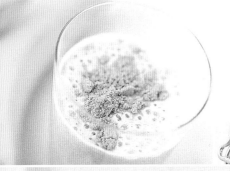

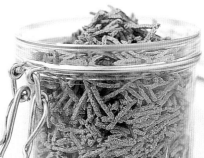

HOW MUCH? A tablespoon of bran provides a sixth of the recommended 30 g of fibre a day. This is similar to the amount of fibre in a slice of wholemeal bread.

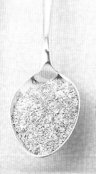
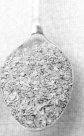
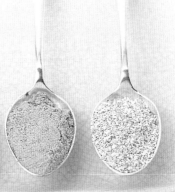

FOOD	CARB	FIBRE	FAT	ENERGY
	g	g	g	kJ
Froot Loops, Kellogg's, 30 g	26.5	0.5	0.5	495
Frosties, Kellogg's, 30 g	27	0.5	0	485
Fruit & Fibre, Weight Watchers, 40 g	31.5	4.5	1	630
Fruit 'n' Nut Weeties, Uncle Tobys, 45 g	31	5	1.5	660
Fruit of the Tropics, 7 am, Willow Valley, 45 g	28.5	4	7	820
Good Start, Sanitarium, 40 g	26	4	2.5	610
Grinners, Honey, Uncle Tobys, 30 g	25.5	3	1	475
Honeycomb Weeties, Uncle Tobys, 30 g	23.5	3	0.5	495
Honey Smacks, Kellogg's, 30 g,	26	1.5	0	490
Just Right, Kellogg's, 45 g	36.5	4.5	1	715
Lite Start, Uncle Tobys, 45 g	35.5	4.5	1	650
MAX NRG, Uncle Tobys, 45 g	36	2	0.5	715
muesli, Apricot & Almond, Morning Sun, 60 g	35.5	8	4.5	880
muesli, Apricot Toasted, Cerola, 30 g	20	4	3	510
muesli, Natural, Sanitarium, 60 g	39.5	4	2.5	875
muesli, Natural, Uncle Tobys, 60 g	35.5	7.5	4.5	880
muesli, Oat 'n Honey Bake, Kellogg's, 45 g	31	5	7	790
muesli, Toasted Tropical, Farmland, 60 g	41	1	8.5	1040
muesli, Toasted Tropical Fruits, Morning Sun, 60 g	40	6	9	1060
muesli, Traditional, Uncle Tobys, 60 g	37	6	4	930
muesli, Weight Watchers, 60 g	44.5	7	4	970
Muesli Flakes, Uncle Tobys, 45 g	32	4.5	1	660
Nut Feast, Uncle Tobys, 45 g	33.5	4.5	3.5	745
Nutrigrain, Kellogg's, 30 g	21.5	1	0	485
Oat Bran, Crunchy, Uncle Tobys, 45 g	30	7	2.5	710
Oat Bran & Fruit, Willow Valley, 40 g	30.5	3.5	3.5	705
Oat Flakes, Uncle Tobys, 30 g	23.5	2	1.5	485
porridge, oat, made with water, 1 cup, 260 g	22	3.5	3	550
porridge, oat, 1/2 water 1/2 whole milk, 1 cup	28.5	2.5	7	870
porridge, oat, 1/2 water 1/2 reduced-fat milk, 1 cup	29.5	2.5	4.5	805
porridge, oat, 1/2 water 1/2 skim milk, 1 cup	28.5	2.5	2.5	740
Puffed Wheat, Sanitarium, 30 g	21.5	2	1	455
Rice Bubbles, Kellogg's, 30 g	26	0.5	0	475
Rice & Oatbran Bubbles, Willow Valley, 30 g	26	1	1	515
Ricies, Fun Bubbles, Sanitarium, 30 g	24.5	0.5	0.5	460
Shredded Wheat, Uncle Tobys, 25 g	18	3.5	0.5	360
Special K, Kellogg's, 30 g	21.5	1	0	480
Sports Plus, Uncle Tobys, 45 g	33.5	3	2.5	730
Sultana Bran, Kellogg's, 45 g	35	6.5	0.5	680
Sultanas 'n' Wheatbran, Uncle Tobys, 45 g	35.5	6.5	1.5	665
Sustain, Kellogg's, 45 g	35.5	3	1.5	715
Vita Brits, Uncle Tobys, 30 g	21	3.5	0.5	435
Weet-bix, Sanitarium, 30 g	19	3.5	1	420
Weet-bix Hi-bran, Sanitarium, 40 g	21	7	3	550
Weet-bix plus Oatbran, Sanitarium, 40 g	26	4.5	1.5	585
Weet-bix, Soy & Linseed, Sanitarium, 40 g	21	7	2.5	520
Wheat Bites, Uncle Tobys, 30 g	25.5	2.5	0.5	475

MUESLI Toasted muesli can be high in fat if it is coated in oil and baked. Natural muesli is lower in fat.

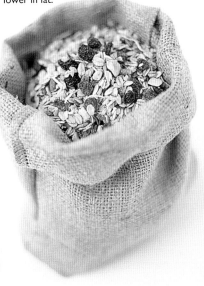

CEREAL Not all breakfast cereals provide a healthy start to the day—many are high in fat, sugar and sodium. However, cereals are a quick and convenient source of energy to power yourself through the morning, and if you check the labels, many provide a low-fat, high-carbohydrate breakfast.

SPORTS CEREALS Advertised as being the ideal way to begin your day, a lot of these are high in sugar, though relatively low in fat.

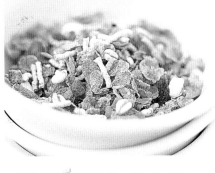

RECIPE If you love toasted muesli, try this low-fat version. Combine 2^1/$_2$ cups rolled oats, ^{1}/$_2$ cup oat bran and 175 g mixed dried fruit and seeds. Drizzle with ^{1}/$_4$ cup maple syrup and bake in a 180°C (350°F/Gas 4) oven for 20 minutes.

WHEAT BISCUITS One of the healthiest ways to start the day. Most contain no sugar, are high in fibre and low in fat.

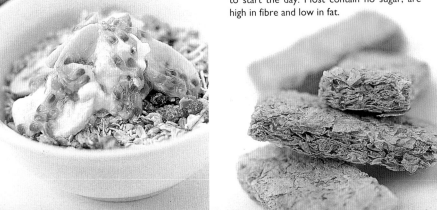

FOOD	CARB	FIBRE	FAT	ENERGY
	g	g	g	kJ
CEREAL BAR (SEE ALSO MUESLI BAR)				
Apricot Fruity Bix Bar, Sanitarium, 1	18	1.5	2.5	440
Lite Start, Uncle Tobys, 1	26	2	2.5	570
Sports Plus, Uncle Tobys, 1	28.5	1.5	2.5	610
CHEESE				
Babybelle, 30 g	0	0	7	375
blue brie, 30 g	0	0	13.5	530
blue castello, 30 g	0	0	10	465
blue vein, 30 g	0	0	9.5	465
bocconcini, 20 g	0	0	7	320
Boursin, 30 g	0	0	10	520
brie, 30 g	0	0	8.5	425
camembert, 30 g	0	0	8	385
canola mild, 30 g	0	0	6.5	395
cheddar, 30 g	0	0	10	505
cheddar, low-fat, Seven, Devondale, 30 g	0	0	7	410
cheddar, processed, 30 g	0	0	8	415
cheddar, reduced-fat, 30 g	0	0	7	410
cheddar slices, Kraft, 20 g	1	0	4.5	255
cheddar slices, reduced-fat, Weight Watchers	1	0	3	200
cheddar sticks, Kraft, 20 g	1	0	6	280
Cheshire, 30 g	0	0	10	480
colby, 30 g	0	0	9.5	485
cottage, 1 tbsp	0	0	2	120
cottage, with cheese, 1 tbsp	0.5	0	0.5	70
cottage, low-fat, Weight Watchers, 1 tbsp	0.5	0	0.5	75
cottage with pineapple, low-fat, 1 tbsp	3	0.5	0	115
creamed cottage, 1 tbsp	0.5	0	1	100
creamed cottage, low-fat, 1 tbsp	1	0	0.5	80
cream, 30 g	1	0	10	425
cream, fruit, 30 g	0	0	7.5	350
cream, light, 30 g	1	0	5	200
cream, Light, Philadelphia, Kraft, 30 g	1	0	4.5	220
cream, low-fat, Neufchatel, Kraft, 30 g	1.5	0	8.5	380
cream, Philadelphia, Kraft, 30 g	0.5	0	10	430
Double Gloucester, 30 g	0	0	10	505
Edam, 30 g	0	0	8	445
emmental, 30 g	0	0	9	475
fetta, 30 g	0	0	7	350
fetta, reduced-fat, 30 g	0	0	4.5	290
goat's, 30 g	0.5	0	4.5	245
Gouda, 30 g	0	0	9	475
halloumi, 30 g	0	0	5	305
havarti, 30 g	0	0	11	505
Jarlsberg, 30 g	0	0	9	475
Jarlsberg Lite, 30 g	0	0	5	340
Lancashire, 30 g	0	0	9.5	465
Leicester, 30 g	0	0	10	500

CHEESE

Whichever way you look at it, cheese is a fairly concentrated source of saturated fat. Although there are reduced-fat brands available, some people find that they taste bland. Do remember that cheese is a good source of calcium and protein and there is no need to cut it out of the diet completely.

PARMESAN Hard cheeses can contain up to 35% fat, but with Parmesan, the strong flavour means that though high in fat, a little can go a long way. Grate with the fine side of the grater and you'll end up using less cheese.

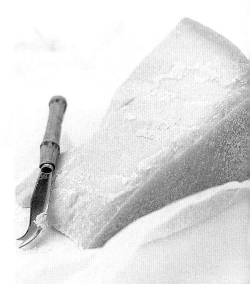

COTTAGE CHEESE The winner in the low-fat competition. Buy the low-fat version and use as a spread, for dips or as a sandwich filling.

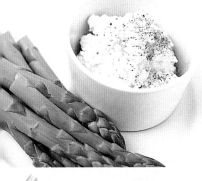

MOZZARELLA Pizza-lovers take note, this cheese is relatively high in fat. If you're making pizza at home, replace half with low-fat mozzarella, so you get lots of taste, but less fat.

RICOTTA Watch out with this cheese, it's not as low-fat as its reputation. A low-fat ricotta is good though: use as a spread, or sweeten with maple syrup for a delicious substitute to cream.

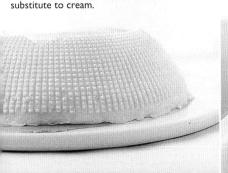

FOOD	CARB	FIBRE	FAT	ENERGY
	g	g	g	kJ
mozzarella, 30 g	0	0	6.5	380
mozzarella, reduced-fat, 30 g	0	0	5.5	360
Parmesan, 30 g	0	0	9.5	555
pecorino, 30 g	0	0	8	445
pepato, 30 g	0	0	9.5	475
pizza, grated, 30 g	0	0	6.5	390
Provolone, 30 g	0	0	8.5	445
quark, 20 g	0	0	2.5	110
quark, low-fat, 20 g	0	0	0.5	65
raclette, 30 g	0	0	9	460
ricotta, 20 g	0	0	2	125
ricotta, reduced-fat, 20 g	0.5	0	1.5	105
Ricotta Smooth, Perfect, 20 g	0	0	2	105
Romano, 30 g	0	0	8.5	470
sheep's milk, Merino Fresh, 30 g	0	0	6.5	380
soy, 30 g	0	0	8	390
Stilton, 30 g	0	0	9.5	465
Swiss, 30 g	0	0	9	480
tilsit, 30 g	0	0	9	465
Wensleydale, 30 g	0	0	9.5	470
CHERRIES				
canned in syrup, drained, 100 g	17	1.5	0	295
glace, 6, 30 g	20	0	0	325
raw, weighed with stones, 100 g	12	1.5	0	225
CHEWING GUM				
sugarless, per piece, 10 g	0	0	0	15
with sugar, per piece, 10 g	3	0	0	40
CHICKEN				
breast, no skin, grilled, 1, 100 g	0	0	5	660
breast, with skin, grilled, 1, 100 g	0	0	12.5	915
breast, quarter, no skin, barbecued, 100 g	0	0	6	835
breast, quarter, with skin, rotisseried, 100 g	1.5	0	12.5	900
Breast, Supreme, Inghams, 1, 100 g	0	0	1	170
Chicken Pastrami, Inghams, 1 serve, 30 g	N/T	N/T	1	170
crispy-skinned, 100 g	0	0	3	270
drumstick, no skin, baked, 2	0	0	9	750
drumstick, with skin, baked. 2	0	0	14.5	960
drumstick, crumbed, 145 g	0	0	17	1315
KFC (SEE FAST FOOD)				
nuggets, 1, 20 g	2.5	0	3.5	240
roll, processed, 1 slice, 38 g	4.5	1.5	9.5	665
sausage, cooked, Steggles, 2	0	0	10	690
spatchcock, baked, 100 g	0	0	14	963
thigh, no skin, cooked, Steggles, 2	0	0	6	530
thigh, with skin, cooked, Steggles, 2	0	0	8	610
wing, with skin, cooked, Steggles, 2	0	0	12	750
CHICKPEAS				
canned, drained, 1 cup, 186 g	24.5	8.5	4	760

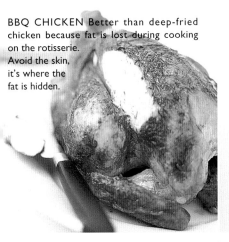

BBQ CHICKEN Better than deep-fried chicken because fat is lost during cooking on the rotisserie. Avoid the skin, it's where the fat is hidden.

CHICKEN A good source of protein and B vitamins. If you are watching the amount of fat in your diet, avoid the skin of the chicken, which makes up about 50% of its fat content (remove it before cooking if possible). Without its skin, chicken is a low-fat source of protein, especially if you poach, steam or grill it.

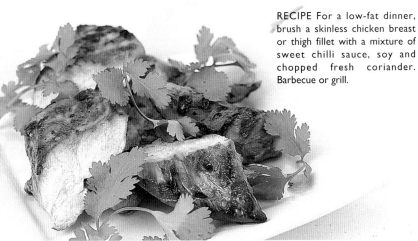

RECIPE For a low-fat dinner, brush a skinless chicken breast or thigh fillet with a mixture of sweet chilli sauce, soy and chopped fresh coriander. Barbecue or grill.

ROAST CHICKEN The juices that come out of a roasting chicken are high in saturated fat. Instead, place on a rack inside a pan and baste with a little oil.

BREASTS VS THIGHS Although chicken breast can be 2 or 3 g lower in fat than the same amount of thigh meat, it tends to dry out if cooked for too long. Thighs are perfect for slower cooking in curries and casseroles.

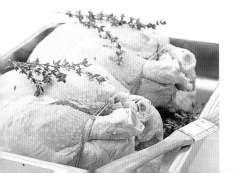

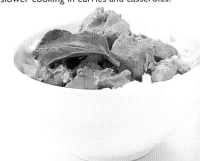

FOOD	CARB	FIBRE	FAT	ENERGY
	g	g	g	kJ
dried, boiled, 1 cup, 180 g	49.5	20.5	4.5	1185
CHICORY GREENS raw, 100 g	1	2	0	50
CHILLI				
banana, raw, each, 80 g	2	1	0	45
green, raw, each, 20 g	0.5	0.5	0	15
red, raw, each, 20 g	1	0.5	0	25
CHIVES fresh, 2 tbsp, 40 g	0	0	0	5
CHOCOLATE				
after-dinner mint, 1, 6 g	11	0	1.5	365
Bounty Bar, Mars, 1, 50 g	30	2.5	12.5	990
Caramello Koala, Cadbury, 1, 20 g	12	0	5.5	415
Cherry Ripe, Cadbury, 1, 55 g	30.5	1.5	13.5	1040
chocolate block, Milka, 100 g	55.5	N/T	32.5	2250
Chocolate Cream, Milka, 100 g	43	N/T	46.5	2535
cooking, dark, Cadbury, 100 g	56	1	31	2120
cooking, dark, Nestlé, 100 g	61.5	1	28.5	2120
Crunchie, Cadbury, 1, 80 g	56	0	16.5	1625
Dairy Milk, Cadbury, 100 g	57	0.5	30	2200
Fantales, Nestlé, 10 individual, 40 g	29.5	N/T	6	710
Fruit & Nut, Nestlé, 100 g	54	2	34	2270
Kit Kat, Nestlé, 1, 45 g	27	N/T	11.5	945
M & M's, milk, Mars, 1 packet, 55 g	40	2	10.5	1080
M & M's, peanut, Mars, 1 packet, 55 g	34	2.5	13.5	1145
Maltesers, Mars, 1 packet, 45 g	30	1	9.5	890
Mars Bar, Mars, 1, 60 g	40.5	1	11.5	1135
Mars Bar, Almond, Mars, 1, 50 g	3.9	1.5	12.5	1150
Milky Bar, Nestlé, 1, 25 g	13.5	0.5	9	575
Milky Way, Mars, 1, 25 g	18	0.5	4	455
Milo Bar, Nestlé, 1, 50 g	N/T	N/T	12	980
Mint Pattie, Nestlé, 1, 20 g	N/T	0	2	330
Picnic, Cadbury, 1, 55 g	27.5	1	16.5	1175
Smarties, Nestlé, 100 g	74	N/T	27	450
Snack, Soft Centres, Cadbury, 100 g	64.5	0	21.5	1970
Snickers, Mars, 1, 60 g	36	1.5	13.5	1190
Time Out, Cadbury, 1, 40 g	23	0.5	11.5	855
Toblerone, 1, 50 g	28.5	N/T	15	1110
Twix, Mars, 1, 55 g	35	1	13.5	1115
Violet Crumble, Nestlé, 1, 50 g	37.5	N/T	9	950
CHOKO (CHAYOTE) 1/2 medium,				
boiled, 85 g	3	1.5	0	70
CHUTNEY				
fruit, 1 tbsp	8.5	0.5	0	145
mango, 1 tbsp	9	0.5	0	125
Cocoa powder 1 tbsp	5	1	3	250
COCONUT				
cream, 1 cup, 250 ml	9	4	50.5	2105
desiccated, dried, 1 tbsp	0.5	1.5	6.5	260
oil, 1 tbsp	0	0	20	740

MILK CHOCOLATE This is usually made by adding milk solids to chocolate. It has the same sugar content as dark and white chocolate.

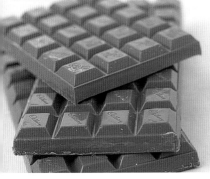

CHOCOLATE Good for an occasional energy boost, a chocolate bar is, however, high in fat and sugar and does contain caffeine. Chocolate is made up of about 30% fat, usually in the form of cocoa butter, and this is what gives chocolate its melt-in-the-mouth texture. Carob is also high in fat, though it is caffeine-free.

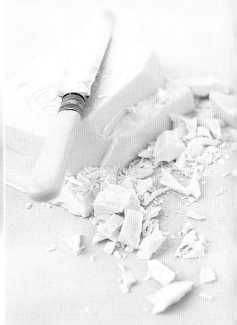

WHITE CHOCOLATE Not a true chocolate because it doesn't contain cocoa solids. It is, however, still made from cocoa butter, milk and sugar and is high in fat.

DARK CHOCOLATE All chocolate is high in fat. However, high-quality chocolate has less sugar, and where this is the case, cocoa solids will come before sugar in the ingredients. Good-quality bitter chocolate has the least sugar.

COCOA The process of manufacturing cocoa powder removes much of the fat content (cocoa butter). Use in cooking to add chocolate flavour without too much fat.

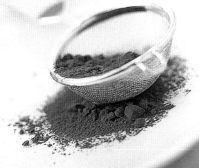

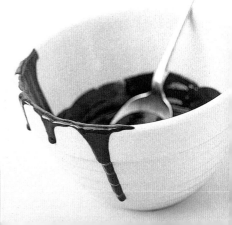

FOOD	CARB g	FIBRE g	FAT g	ENERGY kJ
COFFEE				
for each teaspoon of sugar in coffee, add...	5	0	0	80
cappuccino, whole milk, I cup, 200 ml	N/T	0	5	375
cappuccino, skim milk, I cup, 200 ml	N/T	0	0	210
decaffeinated, black, I cup, 200 ml	0	0	0	8
espresso, black, I cup, 200 ml	4	0	0.5	95
filtered, black, I cup, 200 ml	1.5	0.5	0	30
ground, I cup + 25 ml whole milk, 225 ml	2.5	0.5	1	95
ground, I cup + 25 ml skim milk, 225 ml	2.5	0.5	0	75
iced, plain, I cup, 200 ml	1.5	0	7	250
iced, with whole milk, ice cream & cream, 325 ml	N/T	0	12	750
instant, black, I cup, 200 ml	0	0	0	8
instant, I cup + 25 ml whole milk, 225 ml	1.5	0	1	75
instant, I cup + 25 ml skim milk, 225 ml	1.5	0	0	55
Irish, I cup, 200 ml	N/T	0	10	795
milk, I tsp coffee + I cup whole milk, 200 ml	12.5	1	10	725
mocha, I cup, 200 ml	N/T	0	10	500
percolated, black, I cup, 200 ml	1.5	0.5	0	30
COFFEEMATE whitener, I tsp	2	0	1.5	90
CORDIAL (SEE ALSO SOFT DRINKS)				
citrus, 25% juice, prepared, I glass, 250 ml	17	0	0	275
citrus, 60% juice, prepared, I glass, 250 ml	18	0	0	305
Citrus Twist, Weight Watchers,				
prepared, I glass, 250 ml	N/T	0	0	20
Lemon, Cottees, prepared, I glass, 250 ml	N/T	0	0	290
undiluted, I tbsp	9	0	0	145
CORN				
baby, canned, 6, 100 g	2.5	3.5	0	75
cob, I, 70 g	13	3	0	240
creamed, canned, 100 g	20	4	1	340
kernels, canned, 100 g	18.5	3	1	395
CORN CHIPS (SEE ALSO SNACK FOOD)				
cheese, CC's Original, 40 g	25.5	2	9.5	810
flavoured, 40 g	20	4	12	830
toasted, 40 g	20	11	4	790
CORNMEAL dry, 40 g	30	3	0.5	610
COUSCOUS cooked, 100 g	23	1.5	0	470
CRABAPPLE raw, 60 g	12	1.5	0	190
CRACKERS (SEE ALSO CRISPBREAD)				
Breton, Arnotts, 2	4.5	0.5	2	170
Jatz, Arnotts, 2	5.5	0	1.5	160
Rice Snacks, Cheese, SAN-ESU, 30 g	22	0	2	490
Rice Snacks, Sesame, SAN-ESU, 30 g	22	0	2	490
Ritz, 50% Fat-reduced, Lanes, 2	4	0	1	100
Sao, Arnotts, 2	11	0.5	3	320
Sesame Classic, Lanes, 2	3	0	1	85
Water Crackers, Lanes, 2	4.5	0	0.5	105
CRANBERRY JUICE bottled, I glass, 250 ml	36.5	0.5	0	600

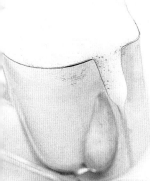

CAPPUCCINOS Skim milk froths up brilliantly for cappuccinos, so there's no reason to add extra kilojoules with whole milk.

COFFEE The French start their day with a café au lait and the Italians survive on espressos, but whichever way you drink your coffee, enjoy in moderation. Caffeine can cause tremors, palpitations and sleeplessness. Milky coffees such as a caffè latte and cappuccino can also be high in fat—choose skim milk if you're watching your kilojoule intake.

STAYING AWAKE A cup of coffee can make you more alert without doing you any harm. However, if you need lots of coffee just to get through the day, then you could look at increasing your intake of carbohydrate-rich foods and doing more exercise to boost your energy levels.

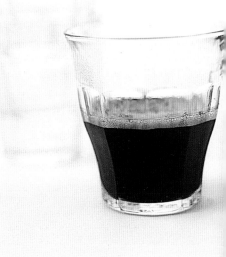

WHICH COFFEE? Instead of ordering a cappuccino or a caffè latte with full-cream milk, try a coffee with skim milk or an espresso.

SUGAR Adding sugar to your coffee will add up to extra kilojoules if you're drinking several cups a day.

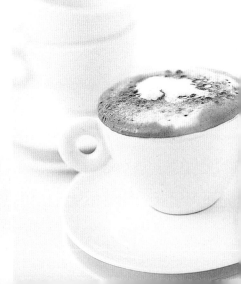

FOOD	CARB	FIBRE	FAT	ENERGY
	g	g	g	kJ
CREAM				
aerosol, whipped, 100 ml	4	0	30.5	1230
clotted, 100 ml	2	0	61	2300
crème fraîche, 100 ml	2.5	0	48	1850
dollop-style, Pauls, 100 ml	2.5	0	35	1390
double thick rich, 100 ml	3	0	54.5	2095
light, 100 ml	3.5	0	17.5	795
regular, 100 ml	3	0	35.5	1400
thickened, 100 ml	3.5	0	36.5	1450
thickened, light, Pauls, 100 ml	6	0	19	885
CREAM, SOUR				
extra light, Pauls, 100 ml	7	0	12.5	665
light, Pauls, 100 ml	5	0	18	810
regular, Dairy Farmer's/Oak, 100 ml	4	0	19	835
CREPE plain, 20 g	7.5	0.5	2.5	275
CRISPBREAD				
CrispKavli, 1, 5 g	4	1	0	70
Cruskits, Bran & Malt, Arnotts, 1	3.5	0.5	0	80
Cruskits, Plain, Arnotts, 1	4.5	0.5	1	115
Cruskits, Rye, Arnotts, 1	4	0.5	0	80
Premium, 97% Fat-free, Lanes, 1	7	0.5	0	145
Premium, Original, Fat-free, Lanes, 1	5	0	1	135
Premium, Wholemeal, Lanes, 1	5	0.5	1	120
Puffed, Rye, Arnotts, 1	4	0.5	0	80
Ryvita, Original, Westons, 1	16	3	0.5	330
Ryvita, Sesame Whole Rye, Westons, 1	15	3	1	340
Salada, Arnotts, 1	10	0.5	1.5	255
Salada, Multigrain, Arnotts, 1	9	0.5	1.5	250
Salada Wholemeal, Arnotts, 1	9	1	1	245
Vita-Wheat, Original, Arnotts, 1	4	1	0.5	95
Vita-Wheat, Original Sandwich, Arnotts, 1	8	1.5	1.5	235
CROISSANT plain, 70 g	25	2	16.5	1150
CROUTONS 1 serve, 15 g	11	1	1	255
CRUMPET				
regular, toasted, 45 g	19.5	1	0.5	390
wholemeal, toasted, 45 g	17	1.5	0.5	355
CUCUMBER				
apple, peeled, 1/4 medium, 80 g	0.5	1	0	25
Lebanese, raw, unpeeled, 5 slices, 35 g	1	0.5	0	15
raw, unpeeled, 5 slices, 45 g	3	0.5	0	15
CUMQUAT raw, peeled, 1, 20 g	3	0	0	50
CURRANTS dried, 1/2 cup, 75 g	49	4 .5	0.5	840
CURRY PASTE				
Green Curry Paste, Mai Thai, 1 tbsp	1.5	N/T	2	100
Indian, Pataks, 1 tbsp	5	0	9	410
Red Curry Paste, Mai Thai, 1 tbsp	1.5	N/T	2	110
Tandoori, 1 tbsp	2	0	0	205

RECIPE For a delicious low-fat alternative to cream, try combining low-fat ricotta with a little low-fat vanilla yoghurt.

THICKENED CREAM Contains about 35% fat. A scoop of low-fat ice cream contains only about 2% fat and would be a healthy alternative to have with dessert.

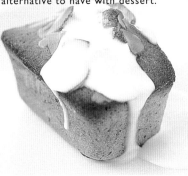

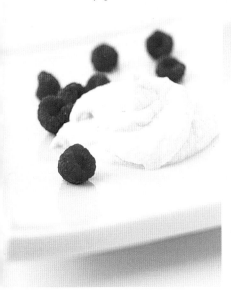

CREAM A concentrated source of saturated fat and cholesterol. However, not all types of cream have the same fat content—the thicker the cream, the more fat it has. Try using light cream or low-fat sour cream, though they are still far from fat-free. An even better alternative is to have your dessert with some low-fat yoghurt or ice cream.

LIGHT CREAM This has about 18% fat—half that of full cream. However, if you use low-fat yoghurt as a substitute, you will reduce the fat level to just 1%.

DOUBLE THICK CREAM Containing about 54% fat, this cream is thick, rich and a very indulgent treat.

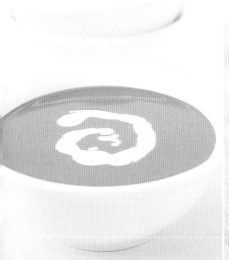

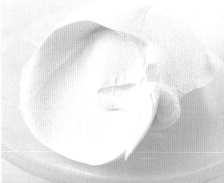

FOOD	CARB	FIBRE	FAT	ENERGY
	g	g	g	kJ
CURRY POWDER 1 tbsp	3	2.5	1.5	125
CUSTARD				
baked, egg, 100 ml	9	0	4.5	400
bread & butter custard, 100 ml	15.5	0.5	5.5	555
Chunky Custard & Fruit, Dairy Vale, 100 ml	16	0	1.5	360
powder, prepared with whole milk, 100 ml	12.5	0	4	405
powder, prepared with reduced-fat milk, 100 ml	13.5	0	1.5	345
pouring, regular, Dairy Vale, 100 ml	16	0	1.5	370
CUSTARD APPLE raw, peeled, 120 g	19	3	0.5	365
DANDELION GREENS raw, 100 g	9	3.5	0.5	190
DANISH PASTRY				
almond, 100 g	46	2	25	1800
Apple, Sara Lee, 100 g	43.5	N/T	12	1250
Apricot, Sara Lee, 100 g	38	N/T	12	1135
Blueberry, Sara Lee, 100 g	40	N/T	12	1200
Chocolate, Sara Lee, 100 g	24	N/T	19.5	1175
Continental, Sara Lee, 100 g	37.5	N/T	17	1365
Custard, Sara Lee, 100 g	34.5	N/T	17	1290
Pecan, Sara Lee, 100 g	52	N/T	20.5	1750
DATES				
dried, 6, 50 g	33.5	5	0	565
fresh, seeded, chopped, 1 tablespoon	25	2.5	0	380
DESSERT				
Apple Pie, Nannas, 100 g	28	N/T	8.5	830
Apple Pie, Sara Lee, 100 g	38.5	N/T	12.5	1170
Apple Pie, Light, Sara Lee, 100 g	32.5	N/T	7	835
Apple Blackberry Pie, Sara Lee, 100 g	42.5	N/T	17	1410
apple & rhubarb crumble, average serve, 120 g	44	3	8	1050
apple strudel, average serve, 100 g	41	2	11	1145
Apricot Pie, Nannas, 100 g	33	N/T	10	975
Apricot Pie, Sara Lee, 100 g	38.5	N/T	14	1230
banana split with 3 scoops ice cream	55	N/T	10.5	1365
Bavarian, Chocolate Mocha, Sara Lee, 100 g	32.5	N/T	23.5	1465
Bavarian, Chocolate Swirl, Sara Lee, 100 g	30.5	0	19.5	1285
Blackberry & Apple Pie, Nannas, 100 g	35	N/T	10	975
Chocolate Mousse, Nannas, 100 g	28	0	13	975
Chocolate Mousse Dessert, Cadbury, 100 g	23	0	9	845
Chocolate Mousse Dessert, Light, Cadbury, 100 g	19	0	4	570
Christmas pudding, average, 1 piece, 50 g	29	2	6	700
custard tart, 1, 135 g	41	1.5	17.5	1470
junket (blancmange), 100 g	18	0	3.5	480
lemon meringue pie, 1 piece, 75 g	28.5	0.5	12.5	1000
Paddle Pop Dessert Log, Streets, 100 g	13	0	6	480
pecan pie, 1 piece, 115 g	64.5	4	21	1890
profiteroles, 1, 55 g	N/T	0	9	545
pudding, Blackberry Sponge, Self-Saucing, White Wings, 165 g	59.5	1.5	5	1255
pudding, bread, 100 g	N/T	N/T	10	1255

BACK-TO-BASICS Home-made rice custard or bread-and-butter pudding made with skim milk make great lower fat desserts. Mum did know best!

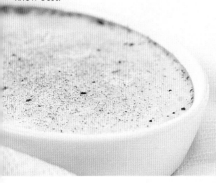

PIES AND TARTS The cream custard varieties tend to be high in fat and kilojoules. Select fruit-based ones if you want less fat.

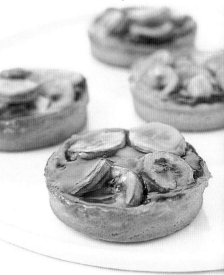

DESSERT

A sweet treat is a perfect way to end a meal, and it doesn't have to be high in fat. A fruit sorbet is a delicious dessert with no fat at all, while pancakes or puddings made with low-fat dairy products are full of energy-giving carbohydrates. Fruit, eaten on its own or with some low-fat yoghurt, is one of the tastiest, and healthiest, desserts of all.

RECIPE Bring 1 cup low-joule cordial, 4 cups water and a cinnamon stick to the boil. Add a peeled pear and simmer for 10–15 minutes until tender. Serve with low-fat fromage frais.

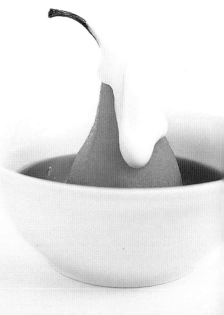

CANNED FRUITS Fruits cooked in their own juice rather than in a sugar syrup are lower in kilojoules.

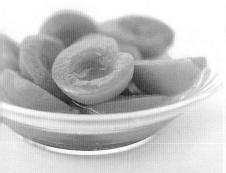

FOOD	CARB g	FIBRE g	FAT g	ENERGY kJ
pudding, Choc Sponge, Puffin, White Wings, 100 g	41.5	N/T	4	910
pudding, Chocolate Mousse, White Wings, 100 g	32	N/T	6	880
pudding, Crème Caramel Royale, White Wings, 100 g	20	N/T	3	500
pudding, Lemon Sponge, Puffin, White Wings, 100 g	41	N/T	3	855
pudding, plum, 1 serve, 60 g	30	1.5	4.5	690
pudding, rice, banana, canned, 1 serve, 125 g	N/T	N/T	13	1025
pudding, rice, chocolate, canned, 1 serve, 125 g	N/T	N/T	6.5	880
pudding, rice, vanilla, canned, Parsons, 150 g	23.5	2.5	2	510
soufflé, 100 g	10.5	0	14.5	840
Tiramisu, 100 g	N/T	N/T	20	1380
trifle, 120 g	33	0.5	7	880
DEVON 2 slices, 50 g	3	0.5	9	490
DIPS				
Barbecue, Kraft, 1 tbsp	2.5	0	4.5	215
Chicken & Asparagus, Dairy Farmers, 1 tbsp	2	0	3	170
Chive & Onion, Kraft, 1 tbsp	1	0	6.5	275
corn'n'bacon, 1 tbsp	2	N/T	1	85
Corn Relish, Dairy Farmers, 1 tbsp	2	0	3	155
French Onion, Dairy Farmers, 1tbsp	1	0	3.5	180
French Onion, Kraft, 1 tbsp	0	0	5	255
French Onion, Light, Kraft, 1 tbsp	3	0	2.5	175
Gherkin Dip, Kraft, 1 tbsp	3	0	4	205
Herb & Garlic, Dairy Farmers, 1 tbsp	2	0	4	190
Hot & Spicy, Dairy Farmers, 1 tbsp	2	0	3.5	185
hummus, 1 tbsp	2	1.5	3.5	190
Salsa, Chilli, Chip'n'Dip, Masterfoods, 1 tbsp	1.5	N/T	0	35
Salsa, Chunky Bean, Chip'n'Dip, Masterfoods, 1 tbsp	2.5	N/T	0	45
taramasalata, 1 tbsp	2	0.5	4	195
tzatziki (cucumber & yoghurt), 1 tbsp	0	0.5	2	110
DOLMADES 60 g	14.5	2.5	4	425
DOUGHNUT				
cinnamon sugar, 1, 50 g	20	1	10.5	770
cream-filled, 1, 70 g	21	0.5	17	1055
iced, 1, 80 g	38.5	1.5	19.5	1425
DRESSINGS (SEE ALSO MAYONNAISE)				
Caesar, Praise, 1 tbsp	3	0	7	320
Caesar, Creamy, Kraft, 1 tbsp	2	0	7	295
Coleslaw, Kraft, 1 tbsp	5	0	7	345
Coleslaw, Praise, 1 tbsp	7	0	7	370
Coleslaw, Light, Praise, 1 tbsp	5.5	0	3.5	240
French, Kraft, 1 tbsp	2.5	0	4.5	205
French, Olive Grove, 1 tbsp	3	0	3.5	180
French, Praise, 1 tbsp	3	0	3.5	180

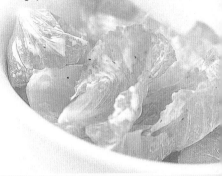

CREAMY DRESSING This can add lots of saturated fat to your salad. For a healthy alternative, combine low-fat yoghurt with orange juice, mustard and herbs.

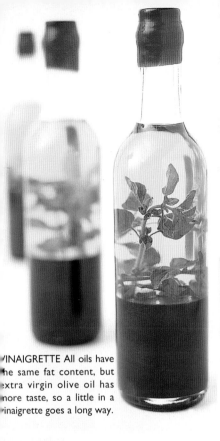

VINAIGRETTE All oils have the same fat content, but extra virgin olive oil has more taste, so a little in a vinaigrette goes a long way.

RECIPE Make a low-fat juice dressing by combining orange juice, mustard, honey and the smallest amount of olive oil.

DRESSINGS A green salad is packed

with fibre, vitamins and minerals, but a heavy hand with the dressing can add lots of unwanted kilojoules. However, the vegetable oils in most dressings do contain the more healthy monounsaturated or polyunsaturated fats, as well as vitamin E. Use more juice or vinegar to oil for a zesty dressing with less fat.

SIMPLE DRESSING Avocados contain quite a lot of fat. Instead of an oily dressing, try just a squeeze of lemon juice and some black pepper.

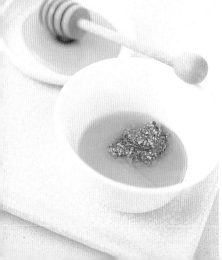

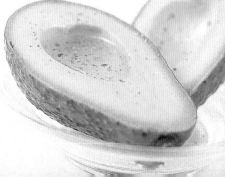

FOOD	CARB	FIBRE	FAT	ENERGY
	g	g	g	kJ
French, Fat-free, Praise, 1 tbsp	3.5	0	0	60
Italian, Kraft, 1 tbsp	1.5	0	6	250
Italian, Olive Grove, 1 tbsp	2	0	3.5	170
Italian, Fat-free, Praise, 1 tbsp	3	0	0	50
Lemon Pepper, Weight Watchers, 1 tbsp	5	0	2	155
Original, Weight Watchers, 1 tbsp	5	0	2	155
Potato Salad, Kraft, 1 tbsp	2.5	0	7	320
Tangy Tomato, Kraft, 1 tbsp	3.5	0	7	320
Thousand Island, Kraft, 1 tbsp	3.5	0	7	320
Thousand Island, Praise, 1 tbsp	3.5	0	4	215
DRINKING POWDER				
Acta-Vite, 1 tbsp	6	0	1	160
Bonox, 1 tbsp	1.5	0	0	100
cocoa, 1 tbsp	1.5	0.5	1	90
Horlicks, 1 tbsp	8	0	0	160
Jarrah, Diet Hot Chocolate Mix, 1 sachet	7	0	1	185
malted milk, 1 tbsp	5.5	0	0.5	135
Milo, Nestlé, 1 tbsp	6	0	1	160
Nesquik, Strawberry, Nestlé, 1 tbsp	12	0	0	210
Ovaltine, 1 tbsp	6	0	0	130
Swiss Miss, Diet Hot Chocolate Mix, 1 sachet	4	0	0	85
DUCK				
roast, no skin, 100 g	0	0	9.5	765
roast, skin, 100 g	0	0	26	1290
EGG				
1 small, 45 g	0	0	4.5	270
1 medium, 55 g	0	0	5.5	325
1 large, 60 g	0	0	6	355
boiled, 1, 53 g	0	0	5.5	335
duck, boiled, 1, 65 g	0.5	0	9	480
Eggs Benedict, 2 eggs	0	1.5	52	2900
fried, 1, 60 g	0	0	8	410
fried, 2 × 60 g, with 1 lean grilled bacon rasher	1	0	19	1055
omelette, plain or herb, 2 × 60 g eggs	0	0	17	900
poached, 1, 60 g	0	0	6	320
poached 2 × 60 g, with 1 lean grilled bacon rasher	1	0	16	990
quail, raw, 1, 10 g	0	0	1	65
replacer, 1 tsp	1.5	0	1	130
scrambled, 2 × 60 g	0.5	0	16	820
turkey, raw, 1, 80 g	1	0	9.5	565
white only, 1, 31 g	0	0	0	60
yolk only, 1, 17 g	0	0	5	225
EGGPLANT				
baby, 4, 65 g	1.5	1.5	0	45
fried in oil, 100 g	2.5	2.5	25	1000
grilled, 3 slices, 90 g	2.5	2.5	0	75
raw, 100 g	2.5	2.5	0.5	75
ELDERBERRIES raw, 1 cup, 145 g	10.5	10	0.5	215

EGG

A good source of protein, vitamins and minerals, eggs have had a hard time because of fears about their high cholesterol level. In fact, to keep your blood cholesterol low, it is more important to avoid saturated fat in your diet. Unless you are watching your cholesterol carefully, eggs can form a nutritious part of everyday eating.

SATURATED FAT Eggs contains about 10% fat, of which under half is saturated. The healthiest way to cook an egg is by boiling or poaching it.

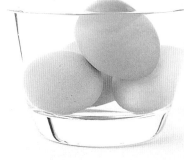

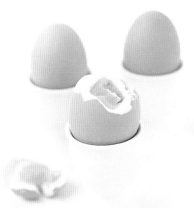

EGG YOLK Very nutritious, but also the source of cholesterol and fat in an egg.

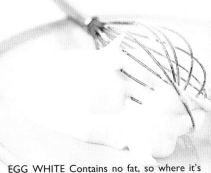

EGG WHITE Contains no fat, so where it's possible, use an egg white rather than the whole egg.

RECIPE Make a more low-fat omelette using one whole egg, 2 egg whites and some skim milk. Mix in fresh herbs and cook without fat in a non-stick pan.

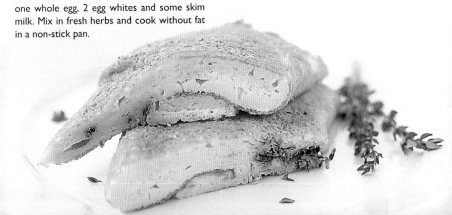

FOOD	CARB	FIBRE	FAT	ENERGY
	g	g	g	kJ
ENDIVE				
Belgian (witlof), raw, 1 cup, 60 g	0	1.5	0	25
curly, 1 cup, 80 g	0	1	0	25
FALAFEL commercial, 2, 60 g	10	7	9	590
FAST FOOD				
battered saveloy, deep-fried, 1, 100 g	18.5	0	21	1280
calamari rings, crumbed & deep-fried, 125 g	15	3	22	1450
chiko roll, 1, 165 g	42.5	2	17	1560
Cornish pastie, 1, 175 g	43.5	2.5	27	1925
dim sim, deep-fried, 1, 50 g	13	0	4.5	465
fish, battered & deep-fried, 1 fillet, 145 g	20	0.5	23	1535
fish stick, crab-flavoured, fried, 1, 27 g	3.5	0	1.5	160
frankfurts, boiled, 2, 100 g	3.5	2	20	1040
hamburger, plain, 1, 170 g	38	3	17.5	1590
hamburger with bacon, 1, 185 g	40.5	3	24	1960
hamburger with cheese, 1, 195 g	41.5	3	26	2105
hamburger with egg, 1, 220 g	44	3.5	26	2170
hot chips, thick, 95 g	25	3.5	13	980
hot chips, thin, 95 g	38.5	3.5	16.5	1290
hot dog, 1, 100 g	18.5	3.5	15	1035
Hungry Jacks, Apple Pie, 1, 80 g	30.5	N/T	13	1005
Hungry Jacks, Bacon Double Cheeseburger Deluxe, 1, 263 g	32.5	25	47.5	2970
Hungry Jacks, Chicken Nuggets, 7, 133 g	17.5	N/T	29.5	1725
Hungry Jacks, Chicken Nuggets, 4, 76 g	10	1	17	990
Hungry Jacks, French Fries, small, 76 g	28.5	N/T	12	950
Hungry Jacks, French Fries, regular, 114 g	42.5	N/T	18	1415
Hungry Jacks, French Fries, large, 159 g	59	N/T	25	1975
Hungry Jacks, Great Aussie Burger, 1, 345 g	55	2.5	32	2715
Hungry Jacks, Grilled Chicken Burger, 1, 180 g	43.5	2	20	2035
Hungry Jacks, Sundae, Caramel/Chocolate, 1, 141 g	36	0	9	1010
Hungry Jacks, Sundae, Strawberry, 1, 141 g	36	0	6.5	915
Hungry Jacks, Thickshake, all flavours, 1, 240 g	48.5	0	8	1255
Hungry Jacks, Whopper, 1, 305 g	52	2.5	38.5	2755
Hungry Jacks, Whopper Junior, 1, 185 g	32	1.5	23.5	1730
KFC, Bacon & Cheese Chicken Fillet Burger, 1, 190 g	34.5	N/T	22.5	1930
KFC, Bacon & Cheese Zinger Burger, 1, 213 g	52	N/T	18.3	2045
KFC, Chicken, Original Recipe, 2 pieces, 154 g	8.5	N/T	29	1735
KFC, Chicken Fillet Burger, 1, 160 g	28	N/T	16.5	1185
KFC, Chips, regular, 117 g	33	N/T	20	1375
KFC, Coleslaw, small tub, 116 g	16	N/T	7	540
KFC, Corn, 1 cobette, 78 g	17	N/T	1	375
KFC, Individual Cheesecake, 75 g	25	N/T	7	735
KFC, Individual Chocolate Mousse, 75 g	17	N/T	5.5	555
KFC, Mashed Potato & Gravy, small tub, 120 g	12.5	N/T	2	335
KFC, Nuggets, 6 pieces, 106 g	18.5	N/T	16.5	1160
KFC, Zinger Burger, 1, 179 g	43.5	N/T	17	1770

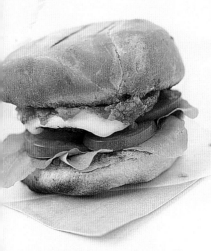

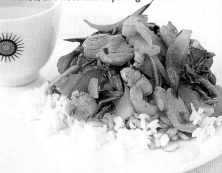

CHINESE Not too bad if you like stir-fries, but deep-fried or battered dishes are fattening. Accompany your meal with steamed rice, not fried, and note that soy is high in sodium.

HAMBURGER This can be nutritious if home-made with lean mince, lettuce and tomato. If you're getting a take-away, skipping the cheese can cut the fat intake by about a third.

MEAT PIES Traditionally high in fat, there are now fat-reduced pies available in supermarkets that have up to 20 g less fat than regular pies.

FAST FOOD Today, more and more people are taking advantage of take-away food. It can be high in fat, but if you look carefully, you'll find there are healthy options. A side dish of vegetables or a salad will fill you up and should be low in fat, while for lunch, the best sandwich choices are turkey or chicken with plenty of lettuce and tomato.

THAI Noodle and some stir-fried dishes are a healthy choice. Avoid curries made with coconut milk as it is high in saturated fat.

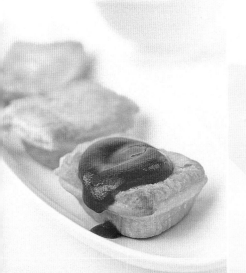

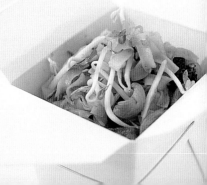

FOOD	CARB	FIBRE	FAT	ENERGY
	g	g	g	kJ
kransky, 1, 80 g	0	0	25	1250
McDonalds, Apple Pie, 1, 85 g	25	3	15	1105
McDonalds, Bacon and Egg McMuffin, 1, 145 g	32.5	2	19.5	1585
McDonalds, Big Breakfast, 1, 250 g	47.5	4.5	31	2385
McDonalds, Big Mac, 1, 205 g	40	2	30	2360
McDonalds, Cheeseburger, 1, 122 g	33	2	12.5	1260
McDonalds, Chicken McNuggets, 9 pieces, 171 g	26	1	26.5	1890
McDonalds, Cookies, 1 box	47	N/T	8.5	1150
McDonalds, Fillet-O-fish, 1, 146 g	40	2.5	16	1475
McDonalds, French Fries, small, 128 g	35	0	16	1200
McDonalds, French Fries, medium	52	4.5	22.5	1740
McDonalds, French Fries, large	65	0	30	2215
McDonalds, Hash Browns, 1, 54 g	15	1.5	7	520
McDonalds, Hot Cakes, with butter & syrup, 1 serve	85	0	15	2010
McDonalds, Junior Burger, 1, 100 g	30	0	10	1120
McDonalds, McChicken, 1, 184 g	46	2.5	20.5	1780
McDonalds, McFeast, 1, 225 g	30	2	3	2100
McDonalds, Quarter Pounder, no cheese, 1, 176 g	36	2	19.5	1750
McDonalds, Sausage Egg McMuffin, 1, 162 g	32	3	22	1730
McDonalds, Sundae, Hot Caramel, 1, 175 g	56.5	0	8	1305
McDonalds, Sundae, Hot Fudge, 1, 175 g	50	0	11	1340
McDonalds, Sundae, Strawberry, 1, 171 g	47	0.5	6	1070
McDonalds, Sundae, without topping, 1, 134 g	29	0	6	770
McDonalds, Thickshake, Chocolate, regular, 1, 305 g	60	1	9.5	1510
McDonalds, Thickshake, Strawberry, large, 1, 419 g	81	0	12.5	2015
Pizza Hut, Pan Pizza, Cheese, 1 slice, 105 g	29	2	10.5	1090
Pizza Hut, Pan Pizza, Hawaiian, 1 slice, 125 g	35	2	11	1225
Pizza Hut, Pan Pizza, Super Supreme, 1 slice, 143 g	35.5	3	15	1425
Pizza Hut, Pan Pizza, Supreme, 1 slice, 136 g	32	3	16	1435
Pizza Hut, Thin'n Crispy, Cheese, 1 slice, 79 g	21.5	1.5	9	910
Pizza Hut, Thin'n Crispy, Hawaiian, 1 slice, 99 g	26	2	9.5	1015
Pizza Hut, Thin'n Crispy, Super Supreme, 1 slice, 117 g	25.5	2.5	14	1215
Pizza Hut, Thin'n Crispy, Supreme, 1 slice, 114 g	27	2.5	12.5	1200
samosa, meat, commercial, heated, 3, 45 g	14	1	9	610
sausage roll, 1, 130 g	31.5	1.5	23	1560
spring roll, deep-fried, 1 large, 175 g	48	2	17	1670

FAT (SEE ALSO BUTTER AND MARGARINE)

cocoa butter, 1 tbsp	0	0	20	740
copha, 1 tbsp	0	0	20	740
dripping, 1 tbsp	0	0	20	740
lard, 1 tbsp	0	0	20	740
replacer, Orgran, 1 tbsp	0	0	0	315
shortening, 1 tbsp	0	0	16	600
suet, 1 tbsp	2	0	17.5	680

FISH AND CHIPS Remember that the thinner the chips, the more surface area and so the more fat is absorbed during frying. Try grilled fish instead of battered. Spring rolls, battered savs and dim sims are all high in saturated fat.

PIZZA Salami, ham and cheese are all high-fat toppings, but any pizza without cheese or meat should be a good choice. If your pizza has a filled base, that'll add kilojoules.

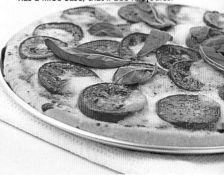

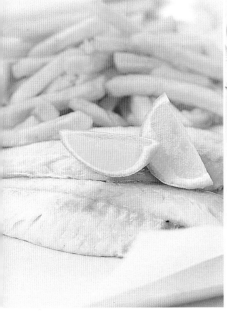

FAST FOOD

The occasional take-away meal or snack is fine if you usually eat a balanced diet. Fast food tends to be short on fresh fruit and vegetables, so a vegetarian pizza or stir-fry would be a good choice, or make up for it later in the day with a low-fat, high-fibre meal that includes an extra portion of vegetables or fruit.

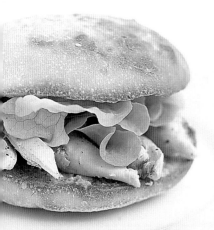

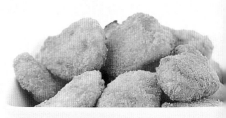

CHICKEN NUGGETS For a low-fat version of these tasty snacks, cut chicken fillets into bite-size pieces, toss in egg white, then coat with cornflake crumbs. Bake in a 200°C (400°F/Gas 6) oven for 10–12 minutes.

SKIN-FREE CHICKEN A lot of the fat in chicken is in the skin, so skin-free chicken is a good choice for a low-fat sandwich or burger.

FOOD	CARB g	FIBRE g	FAT g	ENERGY kJ
FENNEL				
raw, 1 bulb, 150 g	5	4	0	117
steamed, 1 bulb, 150 g	5.5	6	0	130
FIGS				
dried, 5, 75 g	41	10.5	0.5	725
glace, 30 g	N/T	2.5	0	1035
raw, 1, 40 g	3	1	0	70
semi-dried, sweetened, 3, 70 g	34	8	0	325
FISH (SEE SEAFOOD)				
FLOUR				
barley, 100 g	74.5	10	1.5	1445
besan (chickpea), 100 g	58	11	6.5	1545
buckwheat, 100 g	70.5	10	3	1400
cake, 100 g	78	1.5	1	1515
corn, 100 g	91	0	0	1560
maize, 100 g	76	9.5	4	1525
millet, 100 g	75	10	2.5	1525
potato, 100 g	80	2	0.5	1380
rice, 100 g	80.5	2	1.5	1520
rye, wholemeal, 100 g	55	12	2.5	1230
semolina, dry, 100 g	66	3	1	1350
soya, full-fat, 100 g	22.5	12.5	20.5	1720
soya, low-fat, 100 g	25.5	15.5	6.5	1450
triticale, 100 g	73	14.5	2	1415
wheat, white, plain, 100 g	73.5	4	1	1470
wheat, white, self-raising, 100 g	70.5	4	1	1410
wheat, wholemeal, plain, 100 g	52.5	11	2	1170
FRANKFURT				
canned, drained, cooked, 175 g	1.5	1	13	650
cocktail, canned, cooked, 1, 30 g	0.5	0	5	260
cocktail, fresh, cooked, 1, 30 g	1	0.5	6	310
fresh, cooked, 1, 75 g	2.5	1.5	15	780
FRITTATA				
Spanish (potato), 1 slice, 250 g	13.5	1.5	27.5	1550
zucchini & spinach, 1 slice, 250 g	2	2	38.5	1825
FROGS LEGS 2 fried	0	0	10	750
FROMAGE FRAIS				
Fruche, Apricot Honey & Vanilla, 130 g	20	0	0.5	495
Fruche, Orange Tangerine, 130 g	20	0	0.5	505
Fruche, Peach & Mango, 130 g	14.5	0	5	475
Fruche, Strawberry, 130 g	15	0	5	485
Fruche, Strawberry Light, 130 g	18	0	0.5	465
Fruche, Vanilla, 130 g	15	0	5	485
Fruche, Vanilla Light, 130 g	29	0	6	965
Petit Miam, 60 g	10	0	5	365
FROZEN DINNERS				
Beef Goulash, Lean Cuisine, Findus, 400 g	57	N/T	10	1720
Beef Hot-pot, Red Box, McCain, 400 g	39	N/T	11	1495

WHITE FLOUR If you're not a big fan of wholemeal, white flour is still a nutritious alternative and a good protein source.

RICE FLOUR This is a good alternative to wheat flour for anyone with a gluten-intolerance. Maize cornflour, soya and potato flour are also gluten-free.

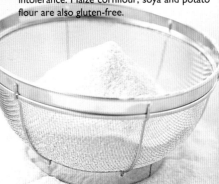

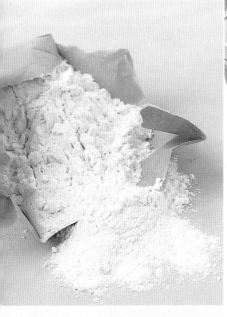

FLOUR
Made into breads, cakes, biscuits and pasta, flour is a good source of carbohydrate. Wholemeal flour is made from the whole grain, while white flour is made after the husk of the grain has been removed and, though still nutritious, does have less fibre, vitamins and minerals. Self-raising flour has more sodium than plain flour.

WHOLEMEAL Full of fibre, vitamins and minerals, wholemeal flour can be used wherever you'd use white flour in cakes, breads, biscuits and pasta-making (you may need to add a little extra water).

SOYA A strong, gluten-free flour that is a richer source of protein than other flours. It can be combined with other flours to make batters and breads.

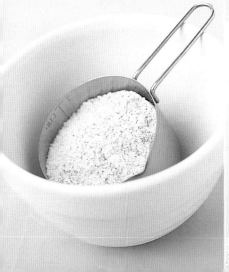

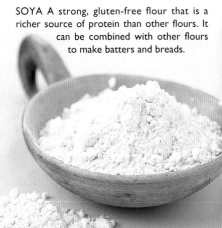

FOOD	CARB	FIBRE	FAT	ENERGY
	g	g	g	kJ
Beef Medallions, Healthy Choice, McCain, 310 g	37	7.5	8	1165
Bubble & Squeak, Birds Eye, per serve	8.5	0	2	215
Chicken Carbonara, Lean Cuisine, Findus, 400 g	76	N/T	11.5	1780
Chicken Chasseur, Healthy Choice, McCain, 310 g	34	6.5	3.5	1055
Chicken Tikka, Healthy Choice, McCain, 400 g	56	N/T	11	1640
Curried Prawns, Red Box, McCain, 350 g	53	N/T	4.6	1255
Fettucine Carbonara, Red Box, McCain, 375 g	49	N/T	30.8	2320
Fettucine Mediterranean, Healthy Choice, McCain, 400 g	58	N/T	11	1660
Fillet of Lamb, Healthy Choice, McCain, 310 g	9	4.5	8	990
Fish Fingers, Birds Eye, grilled, 3, 75 g	15	0.5	7.5	650
French Style Chicken, Lean Cuisine, Findus, 400 g	72	N/T	11.5	2040
Fried Rice, Red Box, McCain, 350 g	20	N/T	7.5	1640
Indian Style Chicken, Lean Cuisine, Findus, 400 g	64	N/T	11	1880
Roast Pork, Healthy Choice, McCain, 320 g	34	N/T	5.5	1165
Satay Lamb, Lean Cuisine, Findus, 400 g	64	N/T	10	1760
shepherd's pie, commercial, 170 g	13.5	1.5	8	745
Thai Style Chicken Curry, Lean Cuisine, Findus, 400 g	64	N/T	12	1840
Veal Cordon Bleu, Healthy Choice, McCain, 320 g	47	N/T	29	2165
FRUCHE (SEE FROMAGE FRAIS)				
FRUIT (SEE INDIVIDUAL FRUITS)				
FRUIT, DRIED (SEE INDIVIDUAL FRUITS)				
FRUIT BAR				
Fruit Fingers, Apricot/Strawberry/Tropical, Heinz, 1 bar, 22 g	15	1.5	0.5	310
Fruit Fingers, Raspberry, Heinz, 1 bar, 15.6 g	13	N/T	0.5	245
Fruit Roll-Up, Uncle Tobys, 1 bar, 37.5 g	23	2	2	680
FRUIT SALAD (SEE ALSO INDIVIDUAL FRUITS AND TWO FRUITS)				
canned in pear juice, drained, 1 cup, 220 g	20.5	3.5	0	385
canned in syrup, drained, 1 cup, 220 g	25.5	2.5	0	445
fresh, 1 cup, 180 g	18	5	0	345
GARLIC				
fresh, 2 peeled cloves, 6 g	0.5	1	0	25
powder, 1 tbsp	7.5	0	0	155
roasted, 6 cloves, 15 g	1.5	3	0.5	65
GELATINE 1 tbsp	0	0	0	175
GHERKINS drained, 36 g	9	1	0	160
GINGER				
beer, dry, 1 cup, 250 ml	22	0	0	345
gingerbread man, 1, 70 g	34.5	0.5	11.5	1045
ground, 1 tbsp	4	0.5	0.5	80
raw, peeled, grated, 1 tbsp	0.5	0	0	15
GNOCCHI potato/pumpkin, average serve, 150 g	13	0	12	895

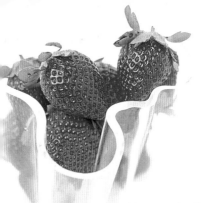

BERRIES A rich source of Vitamin C, all berries contain anitoxidants and they are also low in kilojoules.

FRUIT Packed with vitamins and fibre, nutritionists recommend we eat at least two portions of fruits (and five of vegetables) every day. A portion of fruit is one piece, a cup of berries or a glass of juice. Fruit is a fat-free dessert and is full of antioxidants, which may help to prevent degenerative diseases and even slow down the effects of ageing!

APPLE High in Vitamin C and fibre, apples are also high in fructose, making them a good source of energy.

PAWPAW/PAPAYA Half a medium pawpaw contains lots of beta carotene (an antioxidant) and twice the daily requirement of Vitamin C.

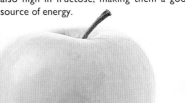

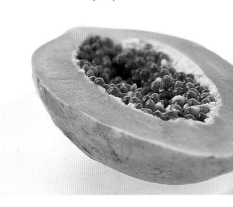

DRIED FRUIT A rich source of dietary fibre, potassium and some iron, but drying destroys the Vitamin C. High in kilojoules, but a good alternative to chocolate for an energy boost.

RECIPE Place some dried fruit in a pan, cover with apple or orange juice and bring to the boil. Stand for 15 minutes until the fruit is plump, then serve warm with low-fat yoghurt.

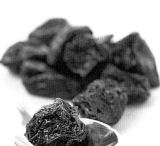

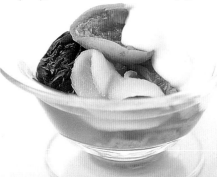

FOOD	CARB g	FIBRE g	FAT g	ENERGY kJ
GOLDEN SYRUP 1 tbsp	21.5	0	0	350
GOOSE lean, roast, 100 g	0	0	23	1325
GOOSEBERRIES				
canned, no added sugar, 100 g	6	2.5	0.5	145
raw, 100 g	9	3.5	0	160
GOURD				
bottle, raw, peeled, 75 g	N/T	2	0	40
ridge, raw, peeled, 75 g	N/T	1.5	0	55
wax, raw, peeled, 75 g	1	1	0	15
GRAPEFRUIT				
canned in juice, 1/2 cup, 125 g	19	0.5	0	330
juice, sweetened, 1 cup, 200 ml	19	0	0	365
juice, unsweetened, 1 cup, 200 ml	16	0	0	300
raw, peeled, 1/2 whole, 110 g	5	1	0	115
GRAPES				
black, 100 g	15	1	0	265
black, muscatel, 100 g	19	1	0	330
green, Cornichon, 100 g	12.5	1	0	235
green, sultana, 100 g	15	1	0	255
juice, sweetened, Berri, 1 cup, 200 ml	N/T	0	1	355
juice, unsweetened, Berri, 1 cup, 200 ml	N/T	0	1	355
Waltham Cross, 100 g	14.5	1	0	255
GRAVY POWDER				
dry, 1 tbsp	8	0	0.5	165
prepared, 1/2 cup, 225 g	3	0	0	60
GUAVA				
canned in juice, 100 g	14.5	3	0.5	260
raw, 1 medium, 100 g	3.5	5.5	0.5	100
HAGGIS boiled, 100 g	150	0.5	20	1220
HALVA 30 g	14.5	0.5	5	430
HAM				
& chicken luncheon meat, 2 slices, 23 g	1	0.5	4	225
light, 90% fat-free, 2 slices, 50 g	0	0	2.5	150
leg, canned, 2 slices, 35 g	0	0	1.5	165
leg, fresh, lean, 2 slices, 46 g	0	0	1.5	210
leg, fresh, untrimmed, 2 slices, 50 g	0	0	4	295
shoulder, 2 slices, 50 g	0	0	3	230
shoulder, canned, 2 slices, 35 g	0	0	2	175
steak, grilled, 1, 115 g	4.5	8.5	9	780
HAMBURGER (SEE FAST FOOD)				
HERBS				
average all varieties, dried, 1 tbsp	0	0	0	80
average all varieties, fresh, chopped, 1 tbsp	0	0	0	70
HONEY 1 tbsp	22	0	0	355
HONEYCOMB 1 piece, 30 g	0	0	1.5	360
HORSERADISH				
Cream, Masterfoods, 1 tbsp	2.5	0	2	135
fresh, 5 g	0.5	0	0.5	35

HERBS

Adding herbs to your food is a healthy way to enhance the flavour of dishes without loading on the fat and salt. Many people also claim that herbs have medicinal properties, and many of today's medical drugs do indeed come from plants. If you are interested in herbal medicine, try some herbal teas, which are now widely available.

BASIL Delicious with tomato dishes and the essential ingredient in pesto, basil is said to have a calming effect and aid digestion. Try basil tea after a rich meal or to relieve nausea.

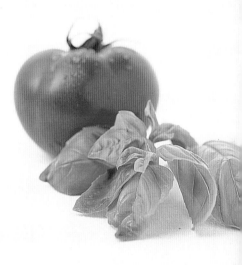

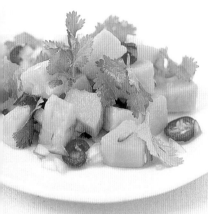

RECIPE Make a healthy fresh salsa from some ginger, pawpaw, chilli, red onion and coriander leaves. Serve with chicken or fish.

ROSEMARY May help to relieve indigestion. To add a subtle rosemary flavour to barbecued meat, tie some rosemary sprigs together and use for basting.

PARSLEY High in vitamins A and C, it is delicious with egg and seafood dishes. Also a great sugarless breath freshener.

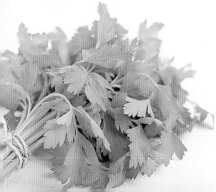

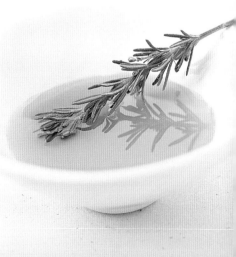

FOOD	CARB g	FIBRE g	FAT g	ENERGY kJ
HUMMUS small serve, 70 g	6.5	6	12	660
ICE BLOCK				
Calippo, Frost, Streets, 1, 158 ml	36.5	0	0	630
Calippo, Lemon, Streets, 100 ml	20	0	0	370
ice confection, tofu, fruit-flavoured, 100 ml	12.5	0	1	280
Icy Pole, Peters, 1, 78 g	16	0	0	270
ICE CREAM				
Caramello Koala Sundae, Cadbury, 1	18	0	6	560
cone, Cornetto, Vanilla, Streets, 1, 70 g	24	0	12.5	925
cone, Cornetto, Chocolate, Streets, 1, 70 g	23	0	13.5	950
cone, Drumstick, Peters, 1, 100 g	24	0	14	990
cone, single, plain wafer type, 1, 15 g	4	0	0	80
cone, sugar, 1, 10 g	8.5	0	0.5	170
cone, waffle, 1, 18 g	3.5	0	0	65
cone with 1 small scoop ice cream, 1	8.5	0	3	270
cone with 1 small scoop reduced-fat ice cream, 1	8.5	0	1.5	225
Crunchie, Cadbury, 1	21	0	19	1090
Freddo, Cadbury, 1	15.5	0	8.5	610
Ranieri, Chocolate, Streets, 100 ml	23	0	11.5	875
Ranieri, Mango, Streets, 100 ml	21	0	8	705
Ranieri, Vanilla, Streets, 100 ml	21	0	10	785
Soft-Serve, McDonalds, 1, 100 ml	21.5	0	4.5	575
Solero, Citrus Lemon, 86 ml	18.5	0	6	575
Solero, Fruits of the Forest, 1, 86 ml	20	0	6	595
stick, Billabong, Chocolate, Peters, 1, 90 ml	19	0	3.5	530
stick, Golden Gaytime, Streets, 1, 75 ml	19.5	0	3	870
stick, Heaven on a Stick, Vanilla, Peters, 1, 93 ml	20.5	0	17.5	1040
stick, Magnum, Classic, Streets, 1, 120 ml	43	0	27	1815
stick, Paddlepop, Chocolate, Streets, 1, 91 ml	18.5	0	8	660
stick, Split, Raspberry, Peters, 1, 90 ml	17.5	0	3.5	450
tub, Blueberry Cream, Peters, 100 ml	10	0.5	5	395
tub, Chocolate, Blue Ribbon, Peters, 100 ml	9.5	0	5.5	385
tub, Cookies & Fudge, Sara Lee, 100 ml	14.5	0	16	905
tub, Honey Malt Marbles, Homer Hudson, 100 ml	N/T	0	18	1220
tub, Light & Creamy Vanilla, Peters, 100 ml	15	0	1.5	325
tub, Natural Vanilla, Peters, 100 ml	10	0	6	425
tub, Original Vanilla, Peters, 100 ml	10	0	4.8	375
tub, Original Extra Creamy Vanilla, Peters, 100 ml	10.5	0	5.5	415
tub, Strawberries & Cream, Sara Lee, 100 ml	22.5	0	10.5	830
tub, Ultra Choc, Sara Lee, 100 ml	21	0	13.5	915
tub, Vanilla Choc Chip, Sara Lee, 100 ml	N/T	0	6	445
tub, Vanilla, Blue Ribbon, Peters, 100 ml	10	0	5	385
tub, Vanilla Light, Blue Ribbon, Peters, 100 ml	12	0	3	350
Viennetta, Chocolate, Streets, 100 ml	13	0	9	559
Viennetta, Toffee, Streets, 100 ml	13	0	10	540
Viennetta, Vanilla , Streets, 100 ml	13	0	10	520
JACKFRUIT raw, peeled, 100 g	17	3	0	320

LOW-FAT FROZEN FRUIT DESSERTS

Sometimes with less than 2 g fat per serving, these desserts are guilt-free and come in a variety of flavours.

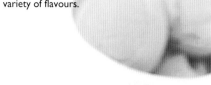

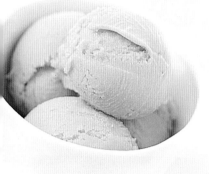

SORBET

With no fat, this is a refreshing, but sweet, alternative to ice cream. Usually made with fruit, so it can be high in vitamin C.

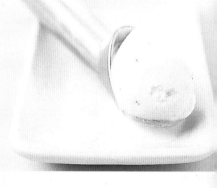

ICE CREAM

As a general rule, the creamier the ice cream is, the higher in fat it is. Ice cream is a good source of vitamins and calcium, but the milk or cream does add saturated fat. There are now many alternatives to ice-cream in our supermarkets, including frozen fruit, tofu or yoghurt desserts—look out for the low-fat varieties.

GOURMET ICE CREAMS

These often contain more fat than ordinary ice creams, but they are made with better-quality ingredients and sometimes contain real fruit.

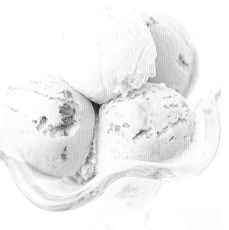

RECIPE

For a tasty and quick dessert, layer a passionfruit fat-free frozen dessert with sliced banana and a spoonful of low-fat honey vanilla yoghurt. Top with some chopped nuts.

FOOD	CARB g	FIBRE g	FAT g	ENERGY kJ
JAM				
average all types, 1 tbsp	17	0.5	0	280
Apricot, Weight Watchers, 1 tbsp	4	0.5	0	70
berry, 1 tbsp	17.5	0.5	0	285
Fruits of the Forest, Weight Watchers, 1 tbsp	4	1	0	70
marmalade, orange, 1 tbsp	17	0	0	275
marmalade, Weight Watchers, 1 tbsp	4	0.5	0	70
JELLY CRYSTALS				
jelly, prepared, 1 cup, 280 ml	45.5	0	0	790
jelly, low-joule, prepared, 1 cup, 270 ml	0	0	0	100
JUICE (SEE INDIVIDUAL FRUITS)				
KALE				
cooked, 1/2 cup, 65 g	3.5	1.5	0.5	75
raw, 35 g	3.5	0.5	0	75
KANGAROO rump, cooked, 100 g	0	0	2.5	430
KIWI FRUIT raw, peeled, 1 small, 75 g	7.5	2.5	0	150
KOHL RABI peeled, boiled, 50 g	2.5	2	0	75
LAMB				
brains, simmered, 80 g	0	0	7.5	450
chump chop, lean, grilled, 1, 55 g	0	0	4.5	465
chump chop, untrimmed, grilled, 1, 65 g	0	0	12	765
cutlet, lean, grilled or baked, 1, 30 g	0	0	4	295
cutlet, untrimmed, grilled or baked, 1, 40 g	0	0	10.5	550
heart, baked, 70 g	0	0	5.5	540
kidney, simmered, 150 g	0	0	6.5	915
leg, lean, baked, 2 slices, 80 g	0	0	5	665
leg, untrimmed, baked, 2 slices, 90 g	0	0	10.5	845
liver, fried, 40 g	0	0	5.5	405
loin chop, lean, grilled, 1, 35 g	0	0	2.5	260
loin chop, untrimmed, grilled, 1, 50 g	0	0	15.5	765
neck chop, lean, stewed, 1, 40 g	0	0	5.5	425
neck chop, untrimmed, stewed, 1, 50 g	0	0	14	740
shank, lean, cooked, 1, 130 g	0	0	4.5	755
shank, untrimmed, cooked, 1, 100 g	0	0	10.5	935
shoulder, lean, baked, 1 slice, 25 g	0	0	2	195
shoulder, untrimmed, baked, 1 slice, 30 g	0	0	6	365
trim, butterfly steak, grilled, 100 g	0	0	4.5	525
trim, fillet, grilled, 100 g	0	0	4	485
trim, roast loin, baked, 100 g	0	0	4	500
trim, schnitzel steak, grilled, 100 g	0	0	3.5	465
trim, strips, grilled, 100 g	0	0	3.5	480
LASAGNE (SEE ALSO PASTA)				
beef, commercial, 400 g	49	12.5	23	2175
Bolognaise, Red Box, McCain, 400 g	67.5	N/T	11.5	2020
Lean Beef Lasagne, Lean Cuisine, Findus, 400 g	64	N/T	8.5	1850
chicken & vegetable, lite, frozen, 1 serve, 300 g	N/T	N/T	0	1260
ricotta & spinach, lite, frozen, 1 serve, 300 g	N/T	N/T	14.5	1260
sheets, dried, 80 g	60	5	2	1180

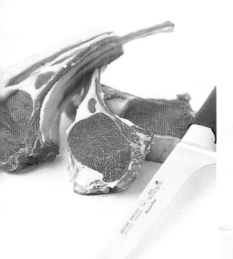

TRIM LAMB For a very lean cut of lamb, try eye of loin or backstrap. Avoid overcooking as lean cuts tend to dry out. Add to a stir-fry or sear on the barbecue instead.

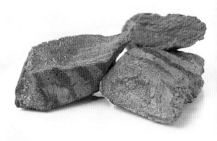

CUTTING FAT OFF LAMB When buying lamb, check how much fat you can see and whether it can be removed—a lamb cutlet that has been trimmed will have a lot less saturated fat. The leanest cuts are the leg and shank, the fattiest the shoulder and rack.

DICED LAMB To make sure your diced lamb is lean, purchase lean cuts such as fillet or eye of loin and dice your own.

LAMB Once thought of as an almost old-fashioned, fatty meat, lamb has come a long way since then. It is no more fatty than beef or pork, and changes in breeding techniques have produced much leaner lambs. Lamb is now on the menu in most good restaurants and there are lots of interesting ways of cooking the new leaner cuts.

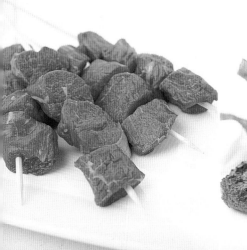

RECIPE For no-fuss, low-fat lamb, marinate trimmed lamb cutlets in tandoori paste, lemon juice and plain low-fat yoghurt overnight. Barbecue until tender.

FOOD	CARB	FIBRE	FAT	ENERGY
	g	g	g	kJ
LECITHIN soy, 1 tbsp	0.5	1.5	6	250
LEEK sliced, boiled, 1/2 cup, 45 g	3	2.5	0.5	85
LEMON				
curd, 1 tbsp	10.5	0	3.5	320
juice, 100 ml	2.5	0	0	110
Flavoured-spread, Kraft, 1 tbsp	13	0	1	250
raw, whole, 1, 65 g	1	1.5	0	60
LENTILS				
burger patty, Vita Burger, Sanitarium,				
1, 70 g	15.5	8.5	1.5	895
dhal, 125 g	14	5.5	9	745
dried, boiled, 200 g	19	7.5	1	590
masurdahl, cooked, 1 cup, 275 g	31	12.5	20	1635
LETTUCE				
cos, 1/2 cup, 35 g	0.5	0.5	0	25
iceberg, 1/2 cup, 35 g	0	0.5	0	10
mignonette, 1/2 cup, 35 g	0.5	0.5	0	20
LIME				
juice, 1 tbsp	2	0	0	25
raw, peeled, whole, 1, 45 g	0.5	1	0	40
LINSEEDS (flaxseeds) 1 tbsp	4	3.5	4	245
LIQUORICE				
allsorts, 5, 50 g	38.5	0.5	2.5	740
pieces, 5, 65 g	4.5	0.5	0	80
LIVERWURST 60 g	0.5	1	17.5	830
LOGANBERRIES raw, 100 g	13	5	0.5	230
LOQUATS 6 medium, 78 g	4	1.5	0	85
LOTUS ROOT				
canned, cooked, 100 g	16	3	0	275
raw, peeled, 100 g	17	5	0	310
LYCHEES				
canned in syrup, drained, 1 cup, 200 g	42.5	3.5	0	730
raw, peeled, 100 g	16	1.5	0	285
MACARONI				
cheese, home-made, 1 cup, 150 g	17	1	22.5	1360
Cheese, Deluxe, Kraft, 1 serve, 243 g	49	2	15.5	1700
Cheese, Traditional, Kraft, 1 serve, 335 g	71	2	21	2340
Cheese & Bacon, Kraft, 1 serve, 293 g	58	2	21	2000
Cheesy Fun Shapes, Kraft, 1 serve, 335 g	71	2	21	2340
plain, boiled, 1 cup, 130 g	37	2.5	0.5	745
MANDARIN				
canned in syrup, drained, 1 cup	36	3	0.5	635
peeled, whole, 1, 60 g	5	1	0	100
MANGO				
canned in syrup, drained, 1 cup	50	2.5	0	845
chutney, 1 tbsp	8.5	0.5	0	145
green, 1/2 cup, 150 g	25	3	0	245
raw, peeled, whole, 1, 150 g	19	2.5	0.5	355

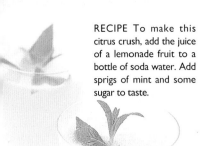

RECIPE To make this citrus crush, add the juice of a lemonade fruit to a bottle of soda water. Add sprigs of mint and some sugar to taste.

LEMON, LIME & ORANGE

Loaded with Vitamin C, just one small orange can meet your whole daily requirement. Vitamin C helps to keep your skin looking healthy and, as an antioxidant, may help to prevent certain diseases. Citrus fruits add flavour to dishes and can be a fat-free way of replacing oils and sweeteners in cooking.

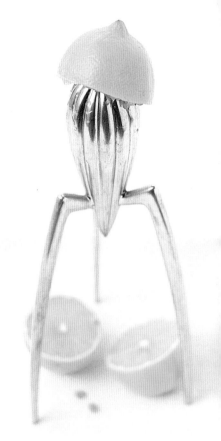

LEMONS Wonderful with fish or in a salad dressing, or try them in a refreshing drink with ice-cold soda water.

ORANGES The whole fruit is better than the juice because the membrane contains fibre. Oranges are also an excellent source of Vitamin C.

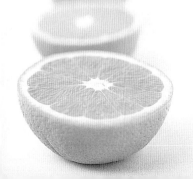

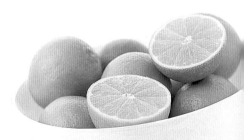

LIMES Delicious with seafood, especially prawns. Limes, like other citrus fruit, contain bioflavonoids that protect the body against free radical damage.

FOOD	CARB	FIBRE	FAT	ENERGY
	g	g	g	kJ
MARGARINE (SEE ALSO BUTTER AND FAT)				
Becel, regular, 1 tsp	0	0	4	155
Becel Light, salt-reduced, 1 tsp	0	0	2	75
Canola Lite, 1 tsp	0	0	3	110
Canola Miracle, 1 tsp	0	0	4	140
Country-Style, Flora, 1 tsp	0	0	4	140
Dairy Blend, Extra-soft, DevonDale, 1 tsp	0	0	3	110
Farmers Blend, Praise, 1 tsp	0	0	3.5	130
Gold'n Canola, Meadow Lea, 1 tsp	0	0	3.5	140
I Can't Believe It's Not Butter, 1 tsp	0	0	4	150
Light, Fat-reduced, Flora, 1 tsp	0	0	2.5	90
Sundew, Meadow Lea, 1 tsp	0	0	4	140
Olive Oil, Olive Grove, 1 tsp	0	0	4	140
Olivio, Bertoli, 1 tsp	0	0	4	140
MARROW				
peeled, boiled, 100 g	4	0.5	0	80
raw, peeled, 100 g	3.5	0.5	0	70
MARZIPAN 20 g	11	1	3.5	335
MATZO				
meal, 50 g	40	1	0	720
plain cracker, 30 g	25	1	0.5	495
MAYONNAISE				
97% Fat Free, Praise, 1 tbsp	9	0	20	190
Cholesterol Free, Kraft, 1 tbsp	7.5	0	3.5	265
Cholesterol Free, Praise, 1 tbsp	7.5	0	7.5	450
Light, Kraft, 1 tbsp	8	0	7	265
Light, Praise, 1 tbsp	7	0	8.5	450
Olive Grove, Meadow Lea, 1 tbsp	5	0	8.5	410
Premium, Kraft, 1 tbsp	7	0	3	245
Traditional, Praise, 1 tbsp	3	0	21.5	845
Weight Watchers, 1 tbsp	7	0	3	230
MEAT SUBSTITUTE (TVP)				
TVP, Sanitarium, 100 g	22	12	2.5	1280
MELON				
casaba, raw, peeled, 100 g	6	1	0	135
honeydew, raw, peeled, 160 g	10.5	1.5	0.5	210
rock, raw, peeled, 250 g	12	2.5	0	230
water, raw, peeled, 100 g	5	0.5	0	95
MERINGUE 25 g	22.5	0	0	385
MILK				
buttermilk, cultured, Dairy Farmers,				
1 cup, 250 ml	4	0	5.5	555
condensed, sweetened, 1 cup, 250 ml	180	0	30	4455
condensed, sweetened, skim,				
1 cup, 250 ml	199	0	1	3785
Contour, Garden City, 1 cup, 250 ml	N/T	0	7.5	440
cultured, reduced-fat, 1 cup, 250 ml	12	0	5	565
cultured, skim, 1 cup, 250 ml	14.5	0	0.5	455

MILK Available in a dazzling number of varieties, milk is the ultimate 'complete food', packed with protein, calcium, vitamins and minerals. Whole milk contains about 4% fat, but for a low-fat alternative, just pick up one of the many reduced-fat or skim milk varieties, which contain almost all the goodness of the whole milk version.

WHOLE MILK Relatively high in saturated fat. It provides essential nutrients, especially for children and pregnant or breastfeeding women.

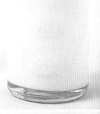

CALCIUM To reach the recommended daily adult intake of calcium, you need to drink three glasses of milk.

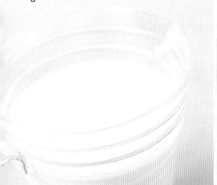

RECIPE For a lactose-free alternative to milk, place almonds or cashews in a blender and process until fine. Add boiling or cold water and a pitted date and blend until smooth. Sprinkle with nutmeg.

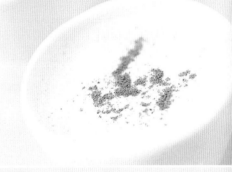

SKIM MILK Except for the loss of Vitamin A, this is just as nutritious as whole milk and can help you control your fat intake.

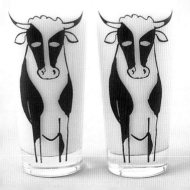

REDUCED-FAT MILK With 50–60% less fat than whole milk, this is a good alternative.

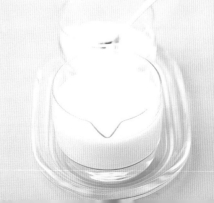

FOOD	CARB	FIBRE	FAT	ENERGY
	g	g	g	kJ
evaporated, reduced-fat, canned, I cup, 250 ml	28.5	0	5.5	1015
evaporated, skimmed, canned, I cup, 250 ml	28.5	0	I	840
evaporated, whole-fat, canned, I cup, 250 ml	27	0	21.5	1565
Farmers Best, I cup, 250 ml	15.5	0	3.5	575
fat-reduced, protein-increased, I cup, 250 ml	14	0	3.5	530
flavoured, chocolate, I cup, 250 ml	23	0	9.5	855
flavoured, chocolate, reduced-fat, I cup, 250 ml	21.5	0	4.5	655
flavoured, Good One, Malt & Honey, Pauls, I cup	27	0	2.5	715
flavoured, strawberry, I cup, 250 ml	23	0	9	845
flavoured, strawberry, reduced-fat, I cup, 250 ml	24	0	4	665
full-cream, I cup, 250 ml	12	0	10	700
goat's, I cup, 250 ml	9.5	0	6.5	535
Lite White, Dairy Farmers, I cup, 250 ml	14.5	0	3.5	558
milkshake, average, 275 ml	47	0	12	1465
milkshake, thick, average, 300 ml	60	0	10	1490
powder, malted, I tbsp	5.5	0	0.5	135
powdered, full-cream, I tbsp	3	0	2	165
powdered, skim, I tbsp	4	0	0	120
Pura Calcium Choice, I cup, 250 ml	12.5	0	2.5	500
Pura Light Choice, I cup, 250 ml	12.5	0	2.5	500
rice, I cup, 250 ml	N/T	0	2.5	660
Shape, fat-free high-calcium, Dairy Farmers, I cup, 250 ml	17	0	0.5	505
sheep's, I cup, 250 ml	13.5	0	17.5	1125
skim, Dairy Farmers, I cup, 250 ml	12.5	0	0.5	370
soy, All Natural, So Natural, I cup, 250 ml	18.5	5	7	665
soy, Life, Pauls, I cup, 250 ml	14.5	0	2.5	475
soy, Life, Low-fat, Pauls, I cup, 250 ml	12	0	1.8	382
soy, Lite, So Good, Sanitarium, I cup, 250 ml	15	0	1.5	450
soy, Now, Soy & Linseed, So Good, Sanitarium, I cup, 250 ml	13	0	8.5	680
soy, Now, Soy & Linseed, Low-fat, So Good, Sanitarium, I cup, 250 ml	13	0	3.8	520
soy, flavoured, Banana Smoothie, So Natural, I cup, 250 ml	23	5	2	580
soy, flavoured, Chocolate Hazelnut, So Natural, I cup, 250 ml	18.5	5	7	665
soy, flavoured, Mango Smoothie, So Natural, I cup, 250 ml	23	5	2	580
soy, flavoured, Utterly Chocolate, So Good, Sanitarium, I cup, 250 ml	20	0	8	750
MILLET cooked, I cup, 174 g	41	2.5	1.5	865
MISO (SOY BEAN PASTE) I tbsp	6	I	I	170
MIXED PEEL 100 g	59	8.5	I	985
MIXED VEGETABLES frozen, boiled, I cup, 145 g	8.5	8.5	0.5	205
MOLASSES I tbsp	14	0	0	225

BUTTERMILK A low-fat alternative to milk, buttermilk has a slightly sour taste and can be used in cooking to replace whole milk.

SOY MILK Not a natural source of calcium, look for low-fat varieties of soy milk with added calcium.

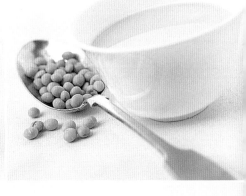

EVAPORATED MILK Simply milk that has had much of its water evaporated. Look for low-fat varieties, which can replace cream in cooking.

MILK
Many people have cut down the amount of dairy products in their diet to limit their fat intake. In fact, it is hard to get enough calcium, which is essential for healthy bones and teeth, from any other source. Switch to low-fat products, and if you have a lactose intolerance, soy milk with added calcium is the best way to meet your calcium needs.

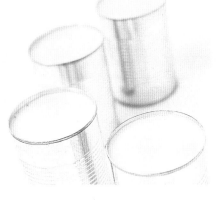

RICE MILK A high-carbohydrate drink, rice milk is a good option for those who are lactose-intolerant. It is sweeter than soy milk.

MILK POWDER Drying milk has little effect on its nutritional value. Use skim-milk powder.

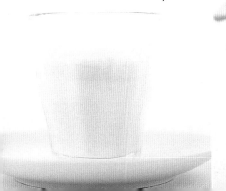

FOOD	CARB g	FIBRE g	FAT g	ENERGY kJ
MUESLI (SEE CEREAL)				
MUESLI BAR (SEE ALSO CEREAL BAR)				
Apricot & Coconut Wrapps, Uncle Tobys,				
1 bar, 31 g	19.5	1.5	7.5	625
Apricot & Fibre, Yoghurt-coated Bar,				
Becoming Healthy, 1 bar, 50 g	28	3.5	9.5	850
Brown Rice Treat, Macadamia & Ginger,				
Wallaby Natural, 1 bar, 50 g	26	1.3	14	985
Chewy Choc Chip, Uncle Tobys, 1 bar, 31 g	21	1.5	5	550
Crunchy Anzac, Uncle Tobys, 1 bar, 31 g	17.5	3	7	615
Crunchy Original, Yoghurt, Uncle Tobys,				
1 bar, 31 g	22	1.5	4	530
Fruit Tops, Apricot, Uncle Tobys, 1 bar, 32 g	22.5	1.5	4.5	575
Nut Crumble, Uncle Tobys, 1 bar, 31 g	20	1.5	6	600
Nut & Muesli, Carob-coated,				
Becoming Healthy, 1 bar, 50 g	28	2	11	915
Peach & Pear, 100 % True Fruit,				
Sun Valley, 1 bar, 25 g	15	0	8.6	550
Yoghurt Tops, Apricot, Uncle Tobys, 1 bar, 31 g	20.5	1.5	5.5	580
Yoghurt Tops, Fruit Salad, Uncle Tobys,				
1 bar, 31 g	21.5	1.5	5	570
MUFFIN				
1 medium, 60 g	29	1.5	8	710
1 large, 100 g	48	2.5	13	1170
1 extra large, 150 g	72	4	19.5	1755
Blueberry, 1, Sara Lee	56	2	13	1480
Bran, Muffin Break, 1, 190 g	67	14	27.5	2310
Calorie-reduced, Muffin Break, 1, 152 g	47.5	6	18	1555
English, Fibre-Increased, Weight Watchers, 1, 63 g	27.5	3.5	2	640
English, fruit, 1, 60 g	27	2	1.5	635
English, Hyfibe, Tip Top, 1	29	4	2	675
English, soy & linseed, 1, 67 g	N/T	N/T	6.5	755
English, Spicy Fruit, Tip Top 1, 67 g	30	2.5	2	705
English, White, Tip Top, 1, 67 g	28.5	2	1	635
English, wholemeal, 1, 67 g	N/T	N/T	2	655
Low-Fat, Muffin Break, 1, 152 g	57.5	10	2.5	1190
Mixed Berry, White Wings, 1, 60 g	38	N/T	5	870
muffin mix, Apple & Sultana, prepared,				
White Wings, 1, 60 g	33	N/T	7	850
muffin mix, Blueberry & Apricot, prepared,				
White Wings, 1, 60 g	32	N/T	6.7	850
muffin mix, Choc Chip, prepared,				
White Wings, 1, 60 g	32	N/T	7	895
MULBERRIES raw, 100 g	4.5	2	0	120
MUSHROOMS				
button, raw, 100 g	1.5	2.5	0.5	100
canned, 100 g	1.5	3	0.5	65
canned in butter sauce, 100 g	3.5	1	1	115

CAROB-COATED BARS An alternative to chocolate, carob has the same amount of fat but is free of caffeine.

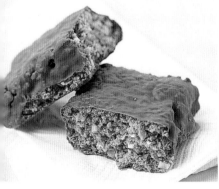

BREAKFAST BARS A good breakfast is a great way to start the day, and these are a convenient alternative to cereal if you're on the run.

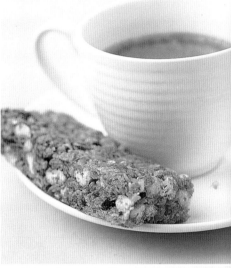

MUESLI & CEREAL BARS Often

eaten as a quick snack or to replace a missed meal, muesli bars can be a good source of dietary fibre and a healthier snack option than a packet of chips or a chocolate bar. However, they are not always as healthy as they seem and can contain up to 17 g fat per bar. Check the label carefully.

MUESLI BARS Some varieties are high in sugar and provide a great energy boost when eaten before or after exercise. If you are not that active, they may provide more energy than you need.

YOGHURT-COATED BARS Handy for a picnic or lunch box, some contain real fruit. Check the fat content on the label.

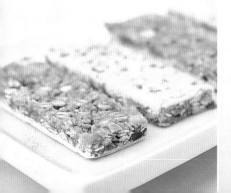

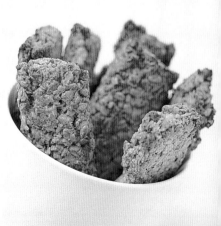

FOOD	CARB	FIBRE	FAT	ENERGY
	g	g	g	kJ
champignon, canned, 1/2 cup, 100 g	I	2	0	55
Chinese, dried & rehydrated, 25 g	4	0	0	60
enoki, raw, 100 g	7	2.5	0.5	145
oyster, raw, 100 g	6	2.5	0.5	155
shiitake, dried, 4, 15 g	II	1.5	0	185
straw, canned, drained, 100 g	4.5	2.5	0.5	135
Swiss brown, 100 g	N/T	4	0	95
MUSTARD				
American, Kraft, 1 tbsp	I	0	0	65
English, Kraft, 1 tbsp	I	0	0	65
French, Kraft, 1 tbsp	I	0	0	65
powder, 10 g	0.5	0	I	75
Seeded, Kraft, 1 tbsp	I	0	0	65
NASHI PEAR raw, unpeeled, 1, 130 g	14	4.5	0	230
NECTARINE raw, unpeeled, 1, 75 g	5.5	2	0	115
NOODLES				
egg, boiled, 1 cup, 100 g	22.5	I	0.5	545
instant, boiled, 1 cup, 100 g	N/T	N/T	5	1540
rice, boiled, 1 cup, 100 g	21.5	0.5	0.5	415
rice, fried, 1 cup, 150 g	27.5	2.5	12.5	1115
rice vermicelli, boiled, 30 g	N/T	N/T	0.5	460
soba (buckwheat), boiled, 100 g	21.5	2	0	415
somen, boiled, 100 g	27.5	I	0	550
Two-minute Noodles, average all flavours, Maggi, 1 packet, 85 g	54	N/T	16	1640
wanton noodles, dry, 100 g	N/T	N/T	3.5	520
wheat, fried, 80 g	50	N/T	17	1570
wheat, steamed, 80 g	60	N/T	2	1190
NUTMEAT canned, Sanitarium, 100 g	6	2	8.5	820
NUTOLENE canned, Sanitarium, 100 g	3	3	18.5	960
NUTS				
almond, blanched, 1/2 cup, 85 g	3.5	7.5	47.5	2110
almond, chocolate-coated, 1/2 cup, 75 g	49.5	4.5	33.5	2170
almond, raw, 4	0.5	1.5	8	365
almond, raw & unpeeled, 1/2 cup, 85 g	4	7.5	46.5	2065
almond, smoked, 30 g	1.5	0	15	815
almond, sugar-coated, 30 g	N/T	0	12	545
Brazil, raw, 1/2 cup, 80 g	2	7	55	2250
bunya, raw, 50 g	35	5	I	350
candle, roasted, 15 g	I	0	10	395
cashew, raw, 1/2 cup, 75 g	12.5	4.5	37	1795
cashew, roasted, 1/2 cup, 75 g	19.5	3	38.5	1970
chestnut, raw, 1/2 cup, 72 g	38	3.5	1.5	735
hazelnut, raw, 1/2 cup, 70 g	3.5	7.5	43	1820
macadamia, raw, 1/2 cup, 73 g	3.5	4.5	55.5	2210
macadamia, roasted, 1/2 cup, 73 g	N/T	I	20	795
mixed, salted, 1/2 cup, 78 g	10	5.5	43	2045
peanut, raw, 1/2 cup, 78 g	7	6.5	36.5	1800

RICE NOODLES A great choice for anyone who can't have wheat in their diet. Cut into strips and add to stir-fries or soups.

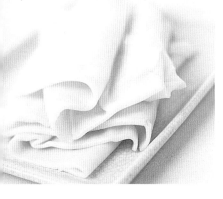

MODERN INSTANT NOODLES These popular wavy-shaped blocks of noodles can be high in fat if they are deep-fried during manufacture.

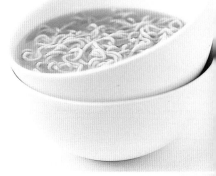

TRADITIONAL INSTANT NOODLES These wheat noodles are steamed, then dried, and so are lower in fat than modern instant noodles.

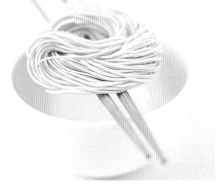

NOODLES
Fast and convenient, noodles are becoming more and more popular, and as the staple of the Japanese diet, they are often seen as a healthy food. Most noodles are high in carbohydrate and low in fat, and when added to soups or stir-fries, make a nutritious meal. Check the labels on instant noodles—they can be high in fat.

HOKKIEN NOODLES Though these fresh egg noodles are tossed in oil before packing, they are used in soups and stir-fries, so are healthier than any crispy fried egg noodles.

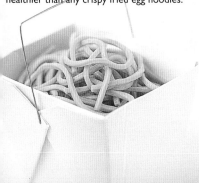

EGG NOODLES Available fresh or dried, avoid them in dishes where they have been fried until crisp, such as in chow mein.

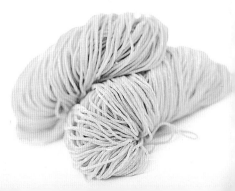

FOOD	CARB	FIBRE	FAT	ENERGY
	g	g	g	kJ
peanut, roasted, 1/2 cup, 78 g	11	5	41	2040
pecan, raw, 1/2 cup, 55 g	2.5	4.5	39.5	1600
pinenut, raw, 1 tbsp, 15 g	0.5	0.5	10	405
pistachio, raw, 1/2 cup, 63 g	4.5	5.5	32	1460
walnut, chopped, raw, 1/2 cup, 55 g	1.5	3.5	38	1570
OATMEAL 40 g	25	3	3	650
OIL				
canola, 1 tbsp	0	0	20	740
cod liver, 1 tbsp	0	0	20	740
olive oil, 1 tbsp	0	0	19	703
vegetable, all varieties, 1 tbsp	0	0	20	740
OKRA boiled, 6 pods, 65 g	1	2.5	0	55
OLIVES				
black, 6 medium, 40 g	2	2	7	165
green, 6 medium, 50 g	2	2	2	125
stuffed, 5 olives, 20 g	0.5	1.5	1.5	75
ONION				
brown, raw, peeled, 1 medium, 100 g	4.5	1.5	0	100
pickled, drained, 2, 36 g	4.5	0.5	0	90
red, raw, peeled, 1 small, 100 g	4.5	1..5	0	105
spring, raw, whole, 1, 14 g	0.5	0.5	0	15
white, raw, peeled, 1 medium, 100 g	4.5	1.5	0	110
ORANGE				
all varieties, raw, peeled, 120 g	9.5	2.5	0	185
juice, commercial, 250 ml	22.5	0.5	0	385
juice, commercial, no added sugar, 250 ml	20	1	0	360
orange & mango juice, 250 ml	20.5	0	0	360
PANCAKE average, home-made, 1, 16 cm, 50 g	14	0.5	1	315
PAPAYA				
green, raw, peeled, 100 g	7	2	0	115
yellow, raw, peeled, 100 g	7	2	0	120
PAPPADUM				
fried, 3 small	N/T	1	2	155
grilled or microwaved, 3 small	N/T	1	0	70
PARSNIP raw, peeled, boiled, 1/2 cup	7.5	2	0	155
PASSIONFRUIT 1 average, 40 g	2.5	6	0	80
PASTA (SEE ALSO LASAGNE AND SPAGHETTI)				
egg, cooked, 1 cup, 200 g	51	2	1	1095
plain, all shapes, cooked, 1 cup, 180 g	44.5	3	0.5	895
Ravioli, Cheese & Spinach, cooked, San Remo, 1 cup, 265 g	88	3.5	16.5	2690
Ravioli, Meat, cooked, San Remo, 1 cup, 265 g	82.5	4	17.5	2530
spinach, cooked, 1 cup, 200 g	54.5	3	1	1085
Soyaroni, cooked, San Remo, 1 cup, 150 g	23.5	2.5	0.5	545
Tomato & Herb Fettucine, cooked, San Remo, 1 cup, 200 g	39	3.5	1.5	780
Tortellini, Cheese & Spinach, cooked, San Remo, 1 cup, 265 g	88	3.5	16.5	2690

RECIPE To make your own basil oil, simply heat some extra virgin olive oil, then add fresh herbs and cool. Process, then strain and use immediately.

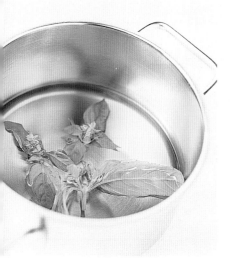

POLYUNSATURATED OILS These oils, such as sunflower or corn oil, contain essential fatty acids that the body cannot produce itself. They may also lower blood cholesterol when they replace saturated fats in the diet.

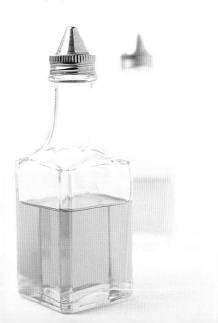

OIL

All oils contain roughly the same amount of fat, but the important issue is what kind of fat? Palm and coconut oils, often used for frying, are high in saturated fat and should be avoided, while the other oils have more monounsaturated and polyunsaturated fats, both of which have health benefits.

MONOUNSATURATED OILS These oils, such as olive, canola or peanut oils, are thought to lower blood cholesterol when they replace saturated fat in the diet.

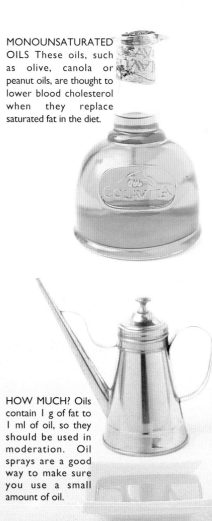

HOW MUCH? Oils contain 1 g of fat to 1 ml of oil, so they should be used in moderation. Oil sprays are a good way to make sure you use a small amount of oil.

FOOD	CARB	FIBRE	FAT	ENERGY
	g	g	g	kJ
Tortellini, Ham & Cheese,				
cooked, San Remo, 1 cup, 265 g	98.5	5.5	15	2765
tortellini, meat, 1 cup	N/T	N/T	5	1590
Vegaroni, cooked, San Remo, 1 cup, 150 g	29.5	2.5	1	590
wholemeal, cooked, 1 cup, 180 g	44.5	10.5	1.5	985
PASTA SAUCE				
Alfredo, San Remo, 1 serve, 125 g	21.5	1	6.5	665
Carbonara, San Remo, 1 serve, 125 g	21.5	1	6.5	665
Creamy Mushroom, Dolmio, 1 serve, 280 g	25	5	0.5	500
Spicy Tomato, San Remo, 1 serve, 125 g	20.5	1.2	5	589
Tomato, bottled, Dolmio, 1 serve, 280 g	26.5	5	2	565
Tomato, Onion & Garlic, bottled,				
Dolmio, 1 serve, 280 g	25	5	0.5	500
PASTRY				
choux, 30 g	7	0.5	8	465
filo, 2 sheets	15	0.5	0.5	325
flaky, average portion, 50 g	21.5	1	14	940
hot-water, 50 g	27	1	10	895
kataifi, 128 g	62	0	12	1600
pizza base, average	N/T	N/T	2	780
puff, 1 sheet, 170 g	60	2	38	2585
shortcrust, 100 g	41	1.5	25.5	1730
strudel, 50 g	23	1	20	1120
suet crust , 50 g	27	1	10	895
wholemeal, 100 g	30.5	7.5	19	1350
PATE				
chicken liver, 1 tbsp	N/T	0	2.5	112
foie gras, 1 tbsp	0.5	0.5	5	250
PAVLOVA				
Pavlova Magic, shell mix, prepared, 1 serve, 60 g	4	0	0	725
shell, with cream & passionfruit, per serve	N/T	3	11	1325
PAWPAW raw, peeled, 100 g	7	2	0	125
PEACH				
canned in jelly, snack pack	N/T	2	0	400
canned in juice, drained, 140 g	12.5	2	0	235
canned, pie filling, 120 g	16	3.5	16	295
canned, snack pack, 140 g	N/T	1.5	0	125
canned in syrup, 250 g	14	2	0	255
dried, 25 g	13	5	0	255
raw, 1 medium, 140 g	9	2	0	185
stewed, with sugar, 100 g	25.5	3	0.5	445
stewed, without sugar, 100 g	21.5	3	0.5	385
PEAR				
canned, snack pack, 140 g	N/T	2.5	0	345
canned in pear juice, drained, 1 cup, 250 g	25.5	4.5	0	445
canned in syrup, drained, 250 g	37	5	0	620
canned in water, drained, 250 g	16	3.5	0	270
dried, 2, 87 g	60.5	6.5	0.5	955

RECIPE For a quick and healthy pasta sauce, cook a chopped onion and garlic clove in a non-stick pan until soft. Add a little red or white wine and some fresh chopped tomatoes and toss together until heated through. Sprinkle with slivers of Parmesan.

CREAMY SAUCES You can make low-fat versions of cream sauces like Alfredo and Carbonara using stock, low-fat milk and some cornflour to thicken.

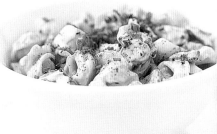

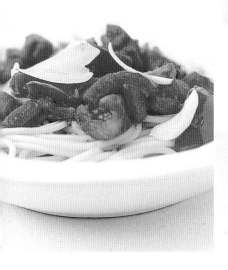

WHOLEMEAL PASTA With over twice the dietary fibre of plain pasta, wholemeal is particularly good in pasta bakes and salads.

PASTA & PASTA SAUCE

High in complex carbohydrates and low in fat, pasta is a great source of energy. To keep the kilojoules down, do as the Italians do, and go easy on the sauce. A home-made tomato pasta sauce is one of the healthiest options, while anything based on cream or cheese is going to have a higher fat content.

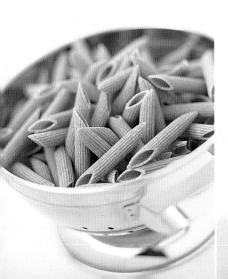

PLAIN PASTA Though the flour used to make plain pasta has had the wheatgerm and bran removed, it still contains plenty of fibre and starch.

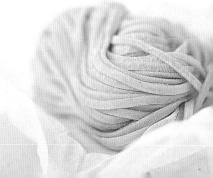

FOOD	CARB g	FIBRE g	FAT g	ENERGY kJ
juice, canned, 200 ml	27.5	0	0	470
raw, unpeeled, 185 g	24	4.5	0	405
PEAS				
green, cooked, 1 cup, 165 g	10.5	10.5	0.5	335
green, frozen, 1 cup, 160 g	9.5	9.5	0.5	335
snowpeas, raw, 170 g	10	7	1	410
split, dried, cooked, 1 cup, 180 g	12	7	1	435
sugar snap, 170 g	10	7	1	410
PEPINO raw, peeled, 1 medium, 120 g	6	1.5	0	110
PERSIMMON raw, peeled, 1 small, 75 g	12	2	0	210
PHEASANT raw, meat only, 125 g	0	0	4.5	695
PIGEON breast, lean, roasted, 125 g	0	0	14.5	1105
PIKELETS Golden, Tip Top, 4, 100 g	28	3	9.5	1110
PINEAPPLE				
canned in juice, drained, 1 cup, 250 ml	25.5	4	0	470
canned in syrup, drained, 1 slice, 40 g	8	0.5	0	140
crushed, canned in juice, drained, 1 cup, 270 g	27.5	4.5	0	510
juice, unsweetened, canned, 250 ml	27	0	0	465
raw, peeled, 1 slice, 110 g	9	2.5	0	175
PIE				
Egg & Bacon, Sara Lee, 100 g	24	N/T	20.5	1325
meat, 1, 190 g	34	2	26	1800
PIZZA				
frozen, Ham & Pineapple, McCain, 1 slice, 100 g	28	N/T	6.5	900
frozen, Perfection, Hawaiian, McCain, 1 slice, 100 g	26	N/T	7.5	910
frozen, Perfection, House Special, McCain, 1 slice, 100 g	23.5	N/T	7.5	895
frozen, Pockets, Ham & Pineapple, McCain, 1 slice, 100 g	33	N/T	8	990
frozen, Pockets, Supreme, McCain, 1 slice, 100 g	30.5	N/T	8.5	995
frozen, Supreme, McCain, 1 slice, 100 g	28.5	N/T	7	935
pizza base, plain, average size, McCain, 235 g	121.5	N/T	8	2735
Pizza Hut (SEE FAST FOOD)				
PLUM				
canned in syrup, drained, 1 cup, 225 g	56.5	5	0.5	955
raw, 100 g	7	2	0	145
stewed, without sugar, 1 cup, 250 g	13	4	0	270
POLENTA dry, 60 g	41	1.5	1	830
POMEGRANATE raw, peeled, 240 g	32.5	15.5	0.5	665
POMELO raw, 100 g	10	0	0	190
POPCORN				
caramel-coated, 100 g	79	5	13	1805
plain, commercial, 2 cups, 16 g	8.5	1.5	4	315
PORK				
bacon, breakfast rasher, grilled, 1, 34 g	0	0	1.5	200
barbecued, Chinese-style, 100 g	3.5	3	15	980
belly, rasher, untrimmed, grilled, 100 g	0	0	22	1250
butterfly steak, lean, grilled, 100 g	0	0	4.5	675

PORK

Thought of as a fatty meat, pork is now bred to be leaner. In fact, lean cuts of pork have less fat than beef, lamb and chicken, and are widely sold under the 'New-fashioned Pork' label. Salami, sausages, spare ribs and bacon are also pork products, but they are higher in saturated fat.

BACON If you love bacon, you can reduce the fat content by up to 50% by trimming off all visible fat and grilling rather than frying.

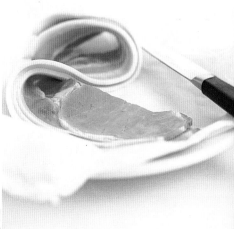

RECIPE To cook lean pork, fry butterfly steaks in a non-stick pan until brown and tender. Remove, then add some sliced apple, wholegrain mustard and apple cider to the pan. Simmer until the apples are soft, add the steaks and reheat.

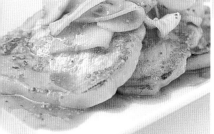

FILLET The leanest cut of pork, this is an excellent substitute for beef or lamb in stir-fries. Alternatively, cut the fillet into slices and grill or barbecue.

BUTTERFLY STEAKS Ideal for filling, these lean steaks are suitable for grilling, pan-frying or barbecuing. Try low-fat fillings such as ricotta and herbs or dried fruit and cooked rice.

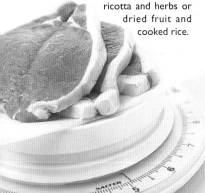

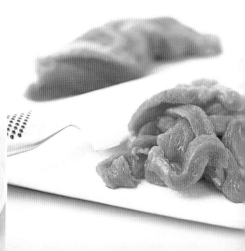

FOOD	CARB g	FIBRE g	FAT g	ENERGY kJ
butterfly steak, untrimmed, grilled, 100 g	0	0	17.5	1090
crackling, 30 g	0	0	9	610
fillet, lean, baked, 1, 100 g	0	0	5	710
forequarter chop, lean, grilled, 1, 95 g	0	0	7.5	720
forequarter chop, untrimmed, grilled, 1, 100 g	0	0	28.5	1440
leg roast, lean, 2 slices, 95 g	0	0	4	685
leg roast, with fat, 2 slices, 100 g	0	0	26.5	1420
leg schnitzel, lean, grilled, 1, 100 g	0	0	3.5	655
leg schnitzel, untrimmed, grilled, 1, 100 g	0	0	6	720
loin chop, lean, grilled, 1, 100 g	0	0	5.5	730
loin chop, untrimmed, grilled, 1, 100 g	0	0	30	1520
medallion steak, lean, grilled, 1 small, 100 g	0	0	5.5	785
medallion steak, untrimmed, grilled, 1 small, 100 g	0	0	22.5	1290
mince, 100 g	0	0	30	1315
pie, 1, 180 g	46.5	2	53.5	3205
ribs, spare, 100 g	0	0	10	480
POTATO				
baked, jacket, no oil, 1 medium, 150 g	21.5	2	1	460
boiled, peeled, 1 medium, 150 g	19.5	1.5	0.5	405
boiled, unpeeled, 1 medium, 150 g	20	2	0	410
canned, peeled, drained, 6 small, 170 g	17.5	2.5	0	355
chips, oven-cook, McCains, 100 g	25	2	3	550
fries (thin-cut), medium serve	43	1	18	1420
gems, oven-fried, 100 g	29	6	13	1030
hash brown, 1 average, 55 g	15	1	12	720
mashed with milk & butter, 1/2 cup, 120 g	N/T	2.5	1	325
mashed with skim milk, 1/2 cup, 120 g	N/T	2.5	0	300
new, peeled, boiled, 3, 165 g	21	3	0	435
roast, no skin, 150 g	26	2.5	4	670
roast, with skin, 150 g	25	2	4	670
scallops, deep-fried, 95 g	26	1.5	20.5	1285
steamed, new, peeled, 165 g	20	3	0	430
wedges, crunchy, McCains, 100 g	26	4.5	6	695
POTATO CRISPS (SEE CORN CHIPS AND SNACK FOOD)				
PRICKLY PEAR raw, peeled, 86 g	7.5	4	0	145
PRUNES				
dried, 5, 38 g	16.5	3	0	295
juice, 250 ml	44.5	2.5	0	760
stewed, with sugar, 150 g	29.5	3	0	500
stewed, without sugar, 150 g	18.5	3.5	0	330
PUMPKIN				
peeled, boiled, 1/2 cup, 85 g	6	1	0.5	150
pie, 1 slice, 109 g	29.5	3	10.5	960
roasted in oil with 1/2 tbsp oil, 85 g	8	1.5	8	525
seeds, dry roasted, 1 tbsp	4.5	1	11.5	565
PURSLANE				
boiled, 1 cup, 115 g	4	N/T	0	85
raw, 1 cup, 43 g	1.5	N/T	0	30

WEDGES For a healthier alternative to chips, lightly spray potato wedges with oil and bake in a 200°C (400°F/Gas 6) oven for 40 minutes until golden.

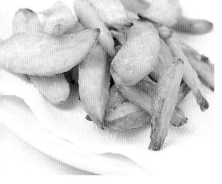

POTATO High in carbohydrate, potassium and Vitamin C, potatoes are a great staple food—it's just the way they're cooked, and their affinity with butter and salt, that can make them unhealthy. Baking is a healthy way to cook potatoes. Boiled potatoes are also low in fat, but Vitamin C is lost in the cooking water.

MASH You can make delicious mashed potatoes without all that butter. Use skim milk or stock, or try adding a little olive oil instead of the butter.

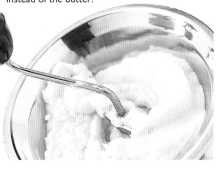

STEAMING A great way to cook potatoes and retain more Vitamin C than boiling. Add some fresh herbs rather than lots of butter and salt.

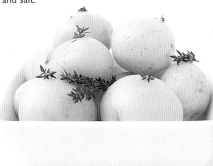

NEW POTATOES There are many potato varieties now available. Make a delicious salad with nutty Pink Fir Apple or Kipfler potatoes and fresh herbs.

FRIES Fried potatoes are all fatty, but the thicker the chip, the less fat is absorbed during cooking. If you love fries, choose wedges.

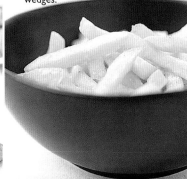

FOOD	CARB	FIBRE	FAT	ENERGY
	g	g	g	kJ
QUAIL				
roasted, with skin, 180 g	0	0	6	755
roasted, without skin, 125 g	0	0	20	1465
QUICHE				
cheese & egg, average home-made, 1 slice, 125 g	21.5	1	27.5	1640
Lorraine, Sara Lee, 100 g	18	N/T	22	1230
Lorraine, mini, Sara Lee, 35 g	7.5	N/T	7	435
mushroom, average home-made, 1 slice, 125 g	23	1.5	24.5	1480
Vegetable, Sara Lee, 100 g	20	N/T	18	1090
Vegetable, mini, Sara Lee, 35 g	8	N/T	6	435
QUINCE				
raw, 100 g	11	7.5	0	200
stewed, with added sugar, 100 g	21	5	0	350
QUINOA grains, boiled, 100 g	69	6	6	1565
RABBIT meat only, baked, 100 g	0	0	5.5	710
RADISH				
red, raw, 3, 45 g	1	0.5	0	2.5
white (daikon), raw, peeled, 1 cup sliced, 90 g	2.5	1.5	0.5	65
RAISINS 100 g	71	5	1	1220
RAMBUTAN raw, peeled, 1, 30 g	5	1	0	85
RASPBERRIES				
canned in syrup, drained, 1/2 cup, 100 g	20	7.5	0	370
raw, 1/2 cup, 65 g	4	3.5	0.5	100
REDCURRANTS raw, 100 g	14	4.5	0	235
RELISH				
corn, 1 tbsp	4.5	0.5	0	85
mustard, 1 tbsp	4.5	0	0	85
tomato, 1 tbsp	4.5	0.5	0	80
RHUBARB				
raw, 100 g	1.5	3	0	75
stewed with sugar, 1/2 cup, 125 g	14.5	2	0	265
RICE				
basmati, cooked, 1 cup	42	N/T	0.3	742
brown, cooked, 1 cup, 180 g	57	3	2	1135
extra-long grain, cooked, Kumamthong, 70 g	54.5	0.5	0.5	973
fried, 1 cup, 190 g	56	2	16	1735
glutinous, cooked, 1 cup, 174 g	36.5	1.5	0	705
jasmine, cooked, Koala Brand, 100 g	34.6	0.5	0.4	651
Sunbrown, cooked, Sun Rice Australia, 100 g	33.4	1.7	1.1	660
Sungold, cooked, Sun Rice Australia, 100 g	34.3	0.8	0.6	653
Sunlong, long grain, cooked, Sun Rice Australia, 100 g	34.6	0.5	0.4	651
Sunwhite, cooked, Sun Rice Australia, 100 g	34.6	0.5	0.4	650
white, cooked, 1 cup, 190 g	53	1.5	0.5	995
wild, cooked, 1 cup, 164 g	35	3	0.5	695
RICE CAKES				
Corn & Buckwheat, Sunfarm, 1, 12 g	10	0.5	0	205
Corn Cakes, Natural, Soy Crisp, Orgran, 2, 10 g	9	1	0	150

RICE The main staple of half the people in the world and an excellent source of energy, rice makes the perfect accompaniment to any meal as it gives a feeling of fullness without adding fat. When mixed with legumes, rice forms a complete protein, which is particularly important for vegetarians. It is also a gluten-free alternative to bread.

RECIPE Next time you make a soup, add some cooked rice to it. It will help to thicken it and raise carbohydrate levels.

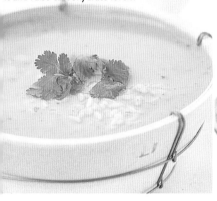

COOKING To maximise the retention of vitamins and minerals, cook rice by the absorption method (follow the manufacturer's instructions).

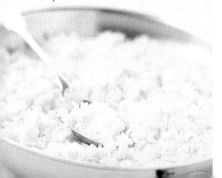

WHITE RICE The bran layer is removed during processing, leaving white rice lower in thiamin than brown rice.

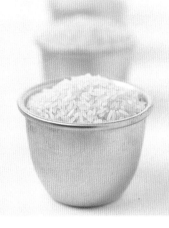

WILD RICE Not a true rice, but a grass native to North America. It can be blended with brown or white rice to add a delicious nutty flavour to dishes.

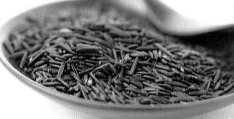

BROWN RICE Definitely the most nutritious choice, it is higher in fibre, vitamins and minerals than white rice.

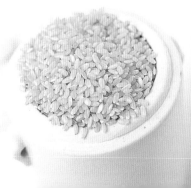

FOOD	CARB	FIBRE	FAT	ENERGY
	g	g	g	kJ
Natural Brown, Sunfarm, 2, 10 g	8	0.5	0.5	160
Rice & Rye, Sunfarm, 2, 10 g	8	0.5	0.5	165
SAFFRON 1 tbsp	1.5	0	0	25
SAGO cooked, 1 cup, 265 g	18.5	1.5	0	315
SALADS				
bean salad, commercial, 1 cup, 210 g	42	8.5	9.5	1105
coleslaw, commercial, 1 cup, 200 g	27	5.5	8	790
potato salad, 1 cup, 180 g	28	1.5	8	815
SALAMI				
average, all varieties, 50 g	0.5	0	19	900
Danish, 4 slices, 20 g	0.5	0.5	8	370
pepperoni, 4 slices, 20 g	0.5	0	7	335
SAPODILLA				
pulp, 1 cup, 241 g	48	12.5	2.5	835
raw, 1, 170 g	34	9	2	590
SAPOTA black, 250 g	58.5	4.5	2.5	975
SAUCES				
aioli mayonnaise, 1 tbsp	0.5	1	13	495
Apricot Chicken, Chicken Tonight, 1 serve, Rosella, 118 g	15	0	1	290
Apricot Chicken, Uncle Ben's, 1 serve, 115 g	16	0	10.5	280
barbecue, 1 tbsp	10	0	0	170
Béarnaise, 1 tbsp	0	0	9	325
Beef & Black Bean, Kan Tong, Masterfoods, 115 g	11	0	1.5	245
bolognaise, 1 cup, 160 g	3.5	1	14	805
butterscotch, 45 g	15	0	17	900
chilli, 20 g	10.5	0	0	40
Country French Chicken, Chicken Tonight, Rosella, 118 g	5	0	11.5	530
Creamy Lemon Chicken, Chicken Tonight, Rosella, 118 g	15	0	0.7	290
Creamy Mushroom & Cracked Pepper, Kan Tong, Masterfoods, 1 serve, 120 g	6.5	0	1.5	560
Creamy Parmigiana, Continental, 120 g	9	0	7	430
Golden Honey Mustard, Chicken Tonight, Rosella, 118 g	12	0	13	715
gravy, commercial, 1/4 cup, 60 g	5.5	0	5.5	340
gravy, made from powder, prepared, 1/4 cup, 60 g	2.5	0	0	60
Herbed Chicken & Wine, Chicken Tonight, Rosella, 1 serve, 115 g	7.5	0	6.5	60
Hoisin, 1 tbsp	7	2	1	170
Honey & Sesame, Continental, 1 serve, 120 g	23	0	1	455
Honey Sesame & Garlic, Kan Tong, Masterfoods, 1 serve, 115 g	23	0	0.5	400
Hungarian Goulash, Continental, 1 serve, 125 g	7.5	0	3.5	440
Malaysian satay, 1 tbsp	5	0.5	5	280
Mild Indian, Kan Tong, Masterfoods, 1 serve, 115 g	8	0	7	390
mint, home-made, 1 tbsp	0	0	0	40

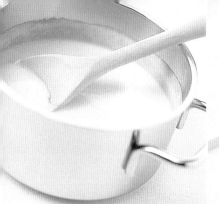

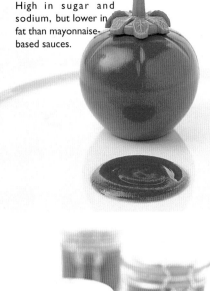

TOMATO SAUCE High in sugar and sodium, but lower in fat than mayonnaise-based sauces.

WHITE SAUCE For a low-fat alternative to this creamy sauce, use skim milk and replace the flour and butter with cornflour.

SAUCES If you are using a small quantity of a sauce like tomato or BBQ, you don't need to worry too much about its nutritional value. Creamy sauces can be very fattening, while Asian sauces are often high in sodium. Where possible, make your own sauces, which will enable you to control the fat, sugar and sodium content.

RECIPE Make your own tomato sauce by simmering some ripe tomatoes, vinegar and a little sugar. Use herbs for added flavour and store in sterilized jars.

COOK-IN SAUCES Can be high in fat and additives, so check the labels. Next time you make a tomato sauce, freeze half so you can add to meat or pasta for an instant dinner.

MINT SAUCE Make your own low-kilojoule version by mixing a handful of chopped mint leaves with a teaspoon each of sugar and boiling water, then stir in 3–4 tablespoons white wine vinegar.

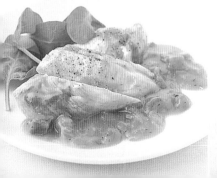

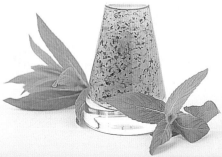

FOOD	CARB g	FIBRE g	FAT g	ENERGY kJ
Mornay Supreme, Continental, 1 serve, 120 g	5	0	14	675
onion, made from powder, prepared, 125 g	8.5	0	7	460
oyster, 1 tbsp	5	0	0	120
packet, average all types, Continental, 1 serve, 125 g	10	0	20	1105
pesto, 1 tbsp	9	1	5	380
Satay, Kan Tong, Masterfoods, 1 serve, 115 g	12.5	0	11	675
soy, 1 tbsp	0.5	0	0	40
Spicy Plum, Kan Tong, Masterfoods, 1 serve, 115 g	21	N/T	0.5	360
Sweet 'n' Sour, Kan Tong, Masterfoods, 1 serve, 115 g	30.5	N/T	0	505
Sweet 'n' Sour Lite, Kan Tong, Masterfoods, 1 serve, 115 g	20.5	N/T	0	335
Sweet Thai Chilli, Kan Tong, Masterfoods, 115 g	52.5	N/T	0.5	855
toffee, 1, 20 g	15	0	2	335
tomato, 1 tbsp	5.5	0.5	0	95
white, home-made, 1 tbsp	2.5	0	5	115
Worcestershire, 1 tbsp	4	0	0	70
SAUSAGE				
beef, fried, home-made, 1, 50 g	2	1	9	490
beef, grilled, home-made, 1, 50 g	3	1	9	535
Bierschinken, 1, 30 g	0	0	5	1300
black pudding, grilled, 1, 90 g	6.5	1.5	21	1180
bratwurst, 100 g	0	0	30	1520
cabanossi, 1, 30 g	0	1	10	460
chicken, thin, 2, 50 g	0	0	6	375
chicken, thin, low-fat, 2, 40 g	0	0	3	295
chipolates (skinless), 2, 25 g	0	0	5	230
chorizo, 1, 60 g	1	0	23	1140
Italian, cooked, 100 g	0	0	30	1520
kransky, 100 g	0	0	35	1560
lap cheong (Chinese sausage), 100 g	3	0	40	1800
low-fat, 1, 50 g	0	0	5	315
mortadella, 1, 30 g	1	0	10	410
pork, thick, grilled, 2, 150 g	9	2	33	1785
pork, thin, grilled, 2, 100 g	6	1.5	21.5	1190
saveloy, 1, 100 g	0	0.5	20	1090
Schinkenwurst, 1, 30 g	0	0	15	645
Vegetarian, Sanitarium, 1, 60 g	4	1	4	410
SCONE				
fruit, 1, 50 g	20	1	3	495
plain, average, 1, 50 g	23	1	5	645
SEAFOOD				
abalone, baked, 85 g	0	0	1	400
anchovies, canned in oil, drained, 5, 18 g	0	0	1.5	140
Balmain bugs, 100 g	0	0	3	500
barramundi, 100 g	0	0	2	390
bass, 100 g	0	0	1	390

TUNA An oily fish, tuna is a good source of Vitamin D and omega-3 fatty acids. Sushi and sashimi are a delicious, low-fat way to consume very fresh fish.

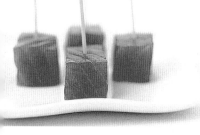

SEAFOOD—FISH

Nutritionists are saying we should eat more fish—but why? Research has shown fish are rich in protein and Vitamin B, while oily fish are the main source of omega-3 fatty acids, which can lower the risk of heart disease and strokes. Low in fat as well, at least two fish meals a week will help towards a healthy diet.

SNAPPER A white fish that is low in fat and high in Vitamin B. It has a subtle flavour and is a good fish to use for steaming, baking or grilling.

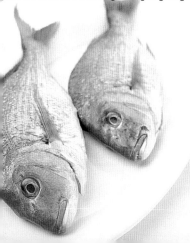

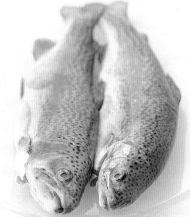

TROUT An oily fish that contains omega-3 fatty acids. It is delicious baked or cooked on the barbecue.

RECIPE For a low-fat dinner, marinate a tuna steak in ginger, lime juice, honey and a little soy for 30 minutes. Chargrill, then serve with steamed rice and stir-fried vegetables.

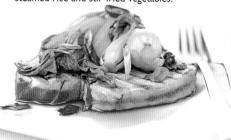

SALMON A well-known oily fish high in omega-3 fatty acids and protein. Salmon is delicious simply poached or baked and served with lemon or dill.

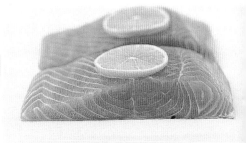

FOOD	CARB g	FIBRE g	FAT g	ENERGY kJ
blackfish, 100 g	0	0	2	390
blue grenadier, 100 g	0	0	2	390
blue threadfin, 100 g	0	0	2	390
boarfish, 100 g	0	0	2	390
bream, steamed, 1 fillet, 149 g	0	0	8	865
calamari tubes, raw, 100 g	0	0	0	290
calamari tubes, fried, 100 g	12	2.5	17.5	1160
caviar, black, 1 tbsp, 16 g	0.5	0	3	170
caviar, red, 1 tbsp, 16 g	0.5	0	3	170
clams, 100 g	0	1	2	340
cockles, raw, 100 g	0	0	0	200
cod, baked, 100 g	0	0	1	320
cod, grilled, 100 g	0	0	2	400
cod, poached, 100 g	0	0	2	400
cod, smoked, simmered, 1 fillet, 195 g	0	0	1.5	375
crab, all varieties, 90 g	0	0	0.5	230
crab, canned in brine, 1 cup, 145 g	2	0	1	370
eel, 85 g	0	0	12.5	800
eel, smoked, 100 g	10	0	13	700
fish ball, boiled, 1, 50 g	2	0	0.5	155
fish paste, 1 tbsp, 20 g	2	0	1.5	130
fish roe, black, 1 tbsp, 20 g	0	0	1	75
fish roe, red, 1 tbsp, 20 g	0	0	1.5	125
fish, steamed, 1 small fillet, 85 g	0	0	2.5	440
flake, crumbed & fried, 1 fillet, 165 g	10.5	0.5	8.5	1230
flake, steamed, 1 fillet, 150 g	0	0	0	785
flathead, fried, 1 fillet, 104 g	3.5	0	7	770
flathead, steamed, 1 fillet, 85 g	0	0	1	405
flounder, 100 g	0	0	1	280
garfish, 100 g	0	0	2	390
gemfish, 1 fillet, 175 g	0	0	27	1650
groper, 100 g	0	0	1	360
gurnard, 100 g	0	0	2	390
haddock, smoked, 1 small fillet, 85 g	0	0	1	35
herring, canned, drained, 125 g	10	0	22.5	1325
jewfish (mulloway), steamed, 1 fillet, 145 g	0	0	4	540
John Dory, 100 g	0	0	1	350
kamaboko, 100 g	0	0	1	220
kingfish, 100 g	0	0	3	440
leatherjacket, 100 g	0	0	2	390
lemon sole, 1 small fillet, 85 g	0	0	2	330
ling, 100 g	0	0	2	390
lobster, boiled, 165 g	0	0	1.5	670
lumpfish roe, 10 g	0	0	1	50
mackerel, 100 g	0	0	16	930
Moreton Bay bugs, 500 g	0	0	3	500
mullet, steamed, 1 fillet, 74 g	0	0	3.5	415
mussels, 100 g	0	0	2	365

SALMON A great cupboard stand-by. Mixed with fresh salad leaves and a squeeze of lemon juice, it makes a healthy light lunch.

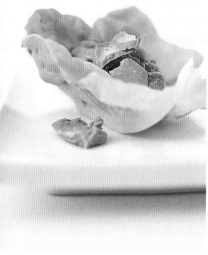

SEAFOOD—CANNED A very convenient way to obtain all the vitamins, minerals and protein of fresh fish. Canning fish does preserve almost all the nutrients, but omega-3 fatty acids may be lost when the fish oil is removed. Canned seafood can be turned into very nutritious quick meals, and is great if you don't have easy access to fresh fish.

RECIPE To make a delicious low-kilojoule sandwich filling, combine canned salmon, chopped spring onion and chives, capers and a squeeze of lemon juice.

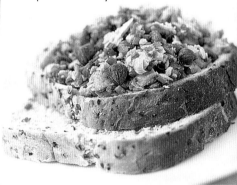

TUNA Select tuna packed in brine or spring water rather than oil. Because the tuna's oil is removed before canning, tinned tuna may have fewer omega-3 fatty acids.

SARDINES Full of protein, iron and zinc. Drain off the oil carefully and pat away any excess that may be left with paper towels.

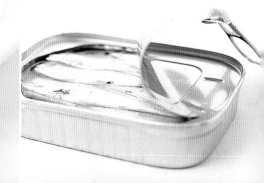

FOOD	CARB	FIBRE	FAT	ENERGY
	g	g	g	kJ
Moreton Bay bugs, 500 g	0	0	3	500
mullet, steamed, 1 fillet, 74 g	0	0	3.5	415
mussels, 100 g	0	0	2	365
mussels, smoked, canned in oil, drained, 100 g	4.5	0	10.5	810
ocean perch, 1 fillet, 120 g	0	0	2.5	470
octopus, 100 g	0	0	1	290
oysters, raw, 10, 60 g	0.5	0	2.5	305
oysters, smoked, canned in oil, drained, 10, 60 g	0.5	0	7	520
parrot fish, 100 g	0	0	2	390
perch, 100 g	0	0	1	360
pike, 100 g	0	0	1	370
pilchards, 150 g	0	0	3.5	660
pilchards, canned in tomato sauce, 225 g	2	0.5	29	1805
prawn cutlets, fried, 3, 75 g	15	1	12	915
prawns, garlic, 100 g	2.5	2	7.5	510
prawns, king, cooked, 100 g	0	0	1	435
prawns, school, steamed, 150 g	0	0	1.5	480
redfish, 100 g	0	0	2	390
salmon, Australian, canned in brine, drained, 100 g	0	0	9.5	720
salmon patty mix, 100 g	0	0	7.5	850
salmon, pink, canned in brine, drained, 100 g	0	0	6.5	615
salmon, raw, 100 g	0	0	12	760
salmon, red, canned in brine, drained, 100 g	0	0	12	815
salmon, roe, 1 tbsp, 10 g	0	0	1	50
salmon, smoked, 50 g	0	0	2.5	280
sardines, fresh, 100 g	0	0	2	280
sardines, canned in oil, drained, 100 g	0	0	15.5	950
sardines, canned in tomato sauce, 100 g	1	0.5	13	800
scallops, steamed, 160 g	1	0	2.5	705
scampi, 100 g	0	0	2	450
scampi, crumbed, fried, 2, 100 g	0	1	17.5	1320
sea bream, 100 g	0	0	5.5	580
sea perch, 100 g	0	0	1	360
sea trout, 100 g	0	0	2	390
shark, 100 g	0	0	1	420
snapper, steamed, 100 g	0	0	2.5	510
sole, 100 g	0	0	1	340
squid, boiled; steamed, 100 g	0	0	1	330
squid rings, fried, 125 g	8.5	0	12	1080
tailor, 100 g	0	0	5	100
teraglin, 100 g	0	0	2	100
trevally, 100 g	0	0	3	440
trout, coral, grilled, 100 g	0	0	2	390
trout, rainbow, steamed, 100 g	0	0	6	650
trout, smoked, 100 g	0	0	5	570
tuna, canned in brine/water, drained, 190 g	0	0	5	985
tuna, canned in oil, drained, 250 g	0	0	28	1890
tuna (sandwich) canned in oil, drained, 100 g	0	0	13.5	920

SELENIUM Shellfish contain the trace mineral selenium, a powerful antioxidant that may protect against disease and have anti-ageing properties.

SEAFOOD—SHELLFISH Though

high in nutrients, shellfish have a reputation for high cholesterol. Cholesterol is present in all animals, and though some shellfish can have a high level, the fact that they are so low in fat, on average less than 2%, means that they are one of the healthiest forms of protein.

RECIPE For a low-fat dinner, marinate peeled raw prawns in garlic, lime juice, macadamia oil and pepper. Barbecue and serve with a low-fat yoghurt and diced watermelon dressing.

OYSTERS Their reputed aphrodisiac quality can be attributed to the fact that oysters have the highest zinc content of any food, a mineral needed for growth and sexual development.

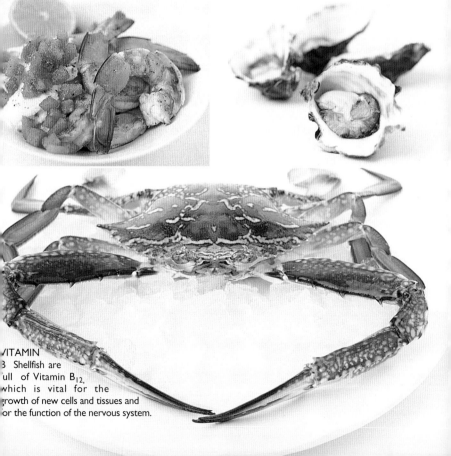

VITAMIN B Shellfish are full of Vitamin B_{12}, which is vital for the growth of new cells and tissues and for the function of the nervous system.

FOOD	CARB	FIBRE	FAT	ENERGY
	g	g	g	kJ
tuna, steamed, 100 g	0	0	3	500
whiting, all varieties, 100 g	0	0	1	390
yabbie, 100 g	1	0	1	300
SEAWEED				
average all types, 10 g	8	0	0	130
SEEDS				
poppy, 1 tbsp	2	1	4	195
pumpkin (pepitas), 50 g	5	12.5	7	650
sesame, 1 tbsp	0	1.5	7	320
sunflower, 1 tbsp	0.5	1.5	8	370
SEMOLINA cooked, 1 cup, 245 g	15.5	1.5	0	315
SHALLOT 25 g	N/T	0.5	0	25
SILVERBEET				
raw, 100 g	1	2.5	0	50
boiled, 100 g	1.5	3.5	0.5	60
SNACK FOOD (SEE ALSO CORN CHIPS)				
Bacon Rings, Sunburst, 1 packet, 25 g	N/T	0	6.5	520
Burger Rings, Smith's, 1 packet, 50 g	0	1	13	1045
Cheese & Bacon Balls, Frito-Lay, 1 packet, 50 g	N/T	N/T	17	1115
Cheese Twisties, Smith's 1 packet, 50 g	30	0.5	13	1045
Cheezels, Smith's, 1 packet, 50 g	30	0.5	15	1085
popcorn, microwave, 1 cup, 100 g	4	1	2	135
potato crisps, plain, 1 packet, 50 g	25	3	15	1045
potato crisps, Kettle Chips, 50 g	N/T	3	16	1050
potato crisps, Lites, 1 packet, 50 g	30	3	15	1085
potato crisps, average all flavours, Pringles, 50 g	N/T	3	18	1185
potato straws, plain, 1 packet, 50 g	N/T	2	17	1085
pork rind, crackling, 1 packet, 30 g	N/T	0	8.5	610
prawn crackers, 5, 30 g	N/T	0	2	190
Pretzels, 10 g	6.5	0.5	0.5	155
sesame seed bar, 1, 45 g	20	3.5	12	700
Toobs, Frito-Lay, 1 packet, 50 g	N/T	N/T	17	1110
SNAIL cooked, 2, 30 g	N/T	0	0.5	120
SOFT DRINKS (SEE ALSO CORDIAL, SPORTS DRINKS AND WATER)				
Coca Cola, 375 ml	39	0	0	630
Coke, Diet, 375 ml	1	0	0	5
dry ginger ale, 375 ml	28	0	0	520
dry ginger ale, diet, 375 ml	1	0	0	15
Fanta, 275 ml	48	0	0	815
Fanta, diet, 375 ml	1	0	0	10
lemonade, 375 ml	40	0	0	670
lemonade, diet, 375 ml	1	0	0	15
Lift, 375 ml	45	0	0	675
Lift, Diet, 375 ml	1	0	0	25
Seven-Up, 375 ml	40	0	0	750
Sprite, 375 ml	40	0	0	630
Sprite, Diet, 375 ml	1	0	0	15
tonic water, 250 ml	0	0	0	345

SOFT DRINKS

The consumption of soft drinks has rapidly increased in the last 20 years, and some of these drinks contain large amounts of sugar, and therefore kilojoules. Small bottles of mineral water are easy to carry around to quench your thirst, while diet sodas are good low-kilojoule alternatives.

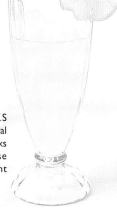

DIET SOFT DRINKS Sweetened with artificial sweeteners, these drinks are suitable for those watching their weight and diabetics.

COLA With 8–10 teaspoons of sugar per can, these drinks are high in kilojoules. Cola also contains significant quantities of caffeine.

FLAVOURED MINERAL WATER These usually have fruit juice added. They can have a comparable sugar content to a glass of cola or lemonade.

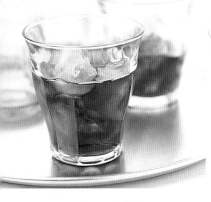

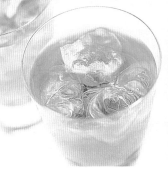

MINERAL WATER The bottles offer a portable alternative to soda for quenching your thirst. Plain sodas and mineral waters are free of kilojoules.

RECIPE Combine pineapple juice, chilled camomile tea and soda water to make a delicious fruit-based soft drink.

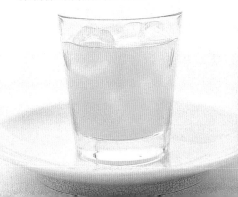

FOOD	CARB g	FIBRE g	FAT g	ENERGY kJ
SORBET lemon, 50 g	7	0	0	260
SOUP				
Chicken, Weight Watchers, 220 ml	8	0.5	1	210
condensed, Beef Broth, Barley				
& Vegetable, Heinz, 220 ml	12.5	0	2.5	340
condensed, Creamy Chicken, Heinz, 220 ml	12	N/T	6	505
condensed, Creamy Chicken & Corn,				
Heinz, 220 ml	14.5	N/T	7	550
condensed, Creamy Chicken & Mushroom,				
Heinz, 220 ml	15	1	0	295
condensed, Creamy Chicken & Vegetable,				
All Natural, Campbells, 215 ml	10.5	N/T	8	585
condensed, Creamy Field-style Mushroom,				
All Natural, Campbells, 215 ml	7	N/T	8	585
condensed, Creamy Golden Pumpkin,				
All Natural, Campbells, 215 ml	13	N/T	4	403
condensed, Creamy Minestrone,				
All Natural, Campbells, 215 ml	15	N/T	0.5	310
condensed, Creamy Potato & Leek,				
All Natural, Campbells, 215 ml	12	N/T	13	755
condensed, Minestrone, Heinz, 220 ml	15	1	0	295
condensed, Mushroom, Heinz, 220 ml	13	N/T	6.5	530
condensed, Pea & Ham, Heinz, 220 ml	15	3	0.5	395
condensed, Salt-Reduced Tomato,				
Heinz, 220 ml	12	2	0.5	240
instant, Chicken Noodle,				
Cup-a-Soup Lite, Continental, 200 ml	5	N/T	0.5	120
instant, Chicken & Vegetable,				
Cup-a-Soup, Continental, 200 ml	14	N/T	0	250
instant, Chunky Southern Chicken,				
Cup-a-Soup, Continental, 250 ml	31	N/T	3	700
instant, Creamy Cauliflower & Cheese,				
Cup-a-Soup Lite, Continental, 200 ml	9	N/T	1	190
instant, Mushroom & Chives,				
Cup-a-Soup Lite, Continental, 200 ml	5.5	N/T	1.5	160
instant, Pea & Ham Supreme,				
Cup-a-Soup Lite, Continental, 200 ml	9.5	N/T	1	230
instant, Pumpkin & Vegetable,				
Cup-a-Soup Lite, Continental, 200 ml	9	0	0.5	170
Minestrone, Weight Watchers, 220 ml	10	2.5	0	210
Tomato, Weight Watchers, 220 ml	11	1.5	0	210
Vegetable, Weight Watchers, 220 ml	9	1.5	0.5	200
SOURSOP (PRICKLY CUSTARD APPLE) raw, 100 g	17	3.5	0.5	275
SPAGHETTI (SEE ALSO PASTA)				
canned, bolognaise, 130 g	12.5	N/T	0.5	285
canned, Tomato Sauce, Heinz, 130 g	16.5	N/T	1.3	365
canned Tomato Sauce & Cheese, Heinz, 130 g	16.5	N/T	1	345
SPICES average all types, 1 tsp	0	0	0	40

SPICES Just like herbs, spices are used in such small quantities that they usually add little nutritional value to our diet. However, adding flavourful and fragrant spices to your food can allow you to use a lighter hand with the salt and cooking oil. Spices have also been renowned for their medicinal properties for centuries.

GINGER May help digestion, and when chewed or made into tea, can be a good relief for morning sickness.

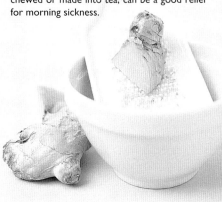

CHILLIS A spicy meal can make the eyes water and the nose run—a good way to bring relief from the blocked airways of a heavy cold.

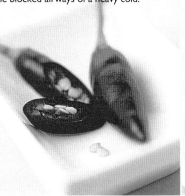

GARLIC A wonder food that contains anti-oxidants and so may boost the immunity system and lower blood pressure.

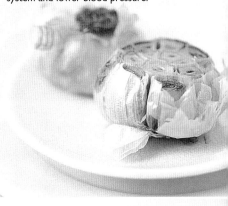

SWEET SPICE Cinnamon, star anise and cardamom are spices that can be used to add flavour to sweet dishes. Infuse in milk, or in a syrup to poach fruit.

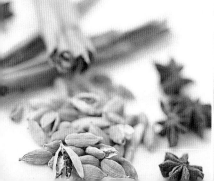

RECIPE For low-fat spicy prawns, marinate peeled and deveined raw prawns in grated ginger, crushed garlic, a finely chopped red chilli and lime juice. Thread onto skewers and barbecue or grill.

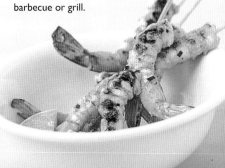

FOOD	CARB	FIBRE	FAT	ENERGY
	g	g	g	kJ
SPINACH				
English, cooked, 35 g	0	2	0	25
English, frozen, 35 g	0	1.5	0	30
English, raw, 35 g	0	1	0	20
SPORTS DRINKS				
Gatorade, 375 ml	22.5	0	0	395
Isosport, 500 ml	36	0	0	630
Isosport Lite, 500 ml	N/T	0	0	605
Lucozade, 300 ml	58	0	0	635
Musashi, 500 ml	N/T	0	0	420
Sport Plus, Schweppes, 500 ml	53	0	0	915
SPREADS (SEE ALSO HONEY AND JAM)				
Almond Spread, 100%, Melrose Natural, 100 g	19	N/T	54	2400
Cheddar Cheese, Kraft, 1 tablespoon	0	0	5	250
Cheddar Cheese, Light, Kraft,				
1 tablespoon	1.5	0	3.5	200
Gherkin, Kraft, 1 tbsp	9.5	5	0	240
Gherkin Sandwich Relish, Kraft, 1 tbsp	10	0.5	0	170
Lemon-flavoured, ETA, 1 tbsp	13	0	1	250
marmalade, orange, 1 tbsp	9	0	0	145
Marmite, Sanitarium, 1 tsp	1	0.5	0	35
Nutella, Ferrero, 1 tbsp	N/T	0	6	440
Peanut Butter, Crunchy, Kraft, 1 tbsp	3.5	0	10.5	525
Peanut Butter, Crunchy Lite, Kraft, 1 tbsp	6	2	7.5	470
Peanut Butter, Smooth, Kraft, 1 tbsp	3.5	0	10.5	525
Peanut Butter, Smooth Lite, Kraft, 1 tbsp	6	2	7.5	470
Pickles, low-joule, Rosella, 1 tbsp	N/T	0	0	35
Promite, Masterfoods, 1 tsp	1.5	0	0	15
Vegemite, Kraft, 1 tsp	0.5	0	0	35
SPRING ONION raw, 12 g	0.5	0	0	10
SPROUTS				
alfalfa seeds, sprouted, raw, 100 g	4	2.5	0.5	120
lentils, sprouted, raw, 100 g	22	N/T	0.5	445
mung beans, sprouted, raw, 100 g	6	2	0	125
radish seeds, sprouted, raw, 100 g	3.5	N/T	2.5	180
soya beans, sprouted, raw, 100 g	9.5	1	6.5	510
wheat seeds, sprouted, raw, 100 g	42.5	1	1.5	830
SQUASH				
button, boiled, 2 whole, 70 g	2.5	2	0	80
scallopini, boiled, 1 large, 70 g	1.5	1.5	0	60
STAR FRUIT (CARAMBOLA) raw, 100 g	12.5	1.5	0	230
STOCK CUBES all varieties, 1, 5 g	1	0	0.5	45
STOCK POWDER all varieties, 1 tbsp	2	0	0.5	80
STRAWBERRIES				
canned in syrup, drained, 1/2 cup, 130 g	24.5	4.5	0	425
raw, 100 g	2.5	2	0	80
STUFFING average, small serve, 30 g	6.5	0.5	2.5	235
SUET MIX 100 g	10	0	90	3390

OTONIC This means that the drink contains the same concentration of carbohydrates as blood, so the carbohydrates can be easily absorbed and blood sugar levels topped up.

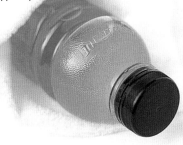

SPORTS DRINKS Lower in sugar than most soft drinks, sports drinks are designed for people who play sport and need a drink that will replace lost fluids and energy rapidly. They contain mineral salts (electrolytes), which are lost through sweating. For more moderate levels of activity, a glass of water or milk is a good choice.

SUGAR Many people drink sports drinks as an alternative to soft drinks as they usually have less sugar.

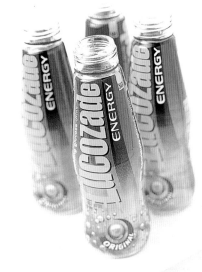

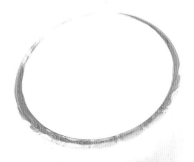

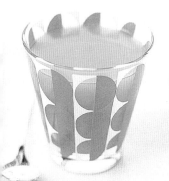

RECIPE Make your own healthy sports drink by combining orange juice, water, a teaspoon of sugar and a small pinch of salt.

SODIUM Sports drinks have added sodium to speed up fluid absorption. Salt lost through perspiration can be replaced through food or even a glass of milk.

FOOD	CARB g	FIBRE g	FAT g	ENERG kJ
SUGAR				
any type, 1 tsp	5	0	0	80
any type, 1 tbsp	17	0	0	270
icing, 1 tbsp	20	0	0	320
SULTANAS dried, 1 tbsp	13.5	0.5	0	230
SUSHI				
Californian Roll, 5 pieces	N/T	N/T	2	585
inari (bean curd pouch with rice), 85 g	N/T	N/T	2	545
nigiri, 30 g	N/T	N/T	0.5	125
SUSTAGEN				
tetra pack, 1, 250 ml	30	5	0	855
Sport, dry, 100 g	65	0	0.5	925
SWEDE (RUTABAGA) peeled, boiled,				
1, 150 g	6	4	0	125
SWEET POTATO				
orange, peeled, boiled, 1, 235 g	33	5.5	0	640
white, peeled, boiled, 1, 235 g	40.5	5	0	750
SWEETS (SEE ALSO CHOCOLATE)				
boiled lollies, 1	5	0	0	65
butterscotch, 1	5.5	0	0	100
caramels, 1	4	0	0	100
clinkers, 1	4.5	0	1	120
fruit gums, 30 g	27	0	0	35
fudge, 2 pieces, 35 g	28.5	0.5	4.5	650
jaffas, 55 g	N/T	0	18	1030
jelly babies, 1	3.5	0	0	65
jelly beans, 1	3	0	0	45
liquorice allsorts, 5, 50 g	38.5	0.5	2.5	740
liquorice pieces, 5, 65 g	4.5	0.5	0	80
Lifesavers, peppermint, 1 packet	N/T	0	0	355
marshmallows, 1 packet, 85 g	68	0	0	1190
sesame seed bar, 45 g	N/T	3.5	12	700
sherbet, lemons, 1	N/T	0	0	85
toffees, 1	3.5	0	0.5	85
SWISS CHARD raw, 1/2 cup, 30 g	1	0.5	0	25
TABOULI 125 g	15	0	15.5	765
TACO with meat & bean sauce, 1 serve, 180 g	N/T	3.5	14	970
TAHINI 1 tbsp	0	2.5	12	520
TAMARILLO (TREE TOMATO) raw, peeled, 90 g	3	4	0	100
TANGELO raw, peeled, 115 g	9	2.5	0	180
TANGERINE raw, peeled, 100 g	5	2	0	100
TAPIOCA cooked, 1 cup, 265 g	18.5	1.5	0	315
TARO peeled, boiled, 100 g	23.5	2.5	0	440
TEA				
for each teaspoon of sugar in tea, add...	5	0	0	80
black, no sugar, 1 cup, 250 ml	0	0	0	5
with whole milk, 1 cup, 250 ml	1	0	1	75
with skim milk, 1 cup, 250 ml	1.5	0	0	55

SUGAR So much focus is now on fat, that many of us forget that we may also eat too much sugar. Sugar provides a burst of energy and causes blood sugar levels to rise quickly, but they fall just as fast. This can result in feelings of hunger, tiredness and irritability. Sugar can also fill us up with 'empty kilojoules'.

HIDDEN SUGAR Much of the sugar in our diet comes from processed food, not from a teaspoon of sugar in our coffee—check the labels carefully.

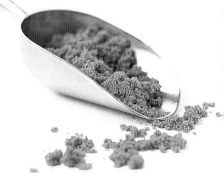

HONEY Although honey and white sugar have about the same amount of kilojoules, honey can be a good substitute, especially as you can use less because of its strong flavour.

SOFT BROWN SUGAR This is in fact white sugar that has been coloured and flavoured with sugar cane molasses. It has no nutritional benefits over white sugar.

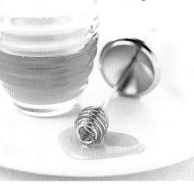

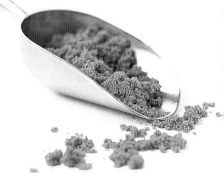

ARTIFICIAL SUGARS These contain no kilojoules and offer a sugar substitute for people cutting down their sugar intake.

MAPLE SYRUP Made from the sap of the maple tree, this syrup is an alternative to sugar.

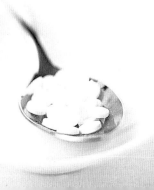

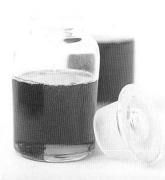

FOOD	CARB g	FIBRE g	FAT g	ENERG kJ
TEMPEH				
burger, grilled, 43 g	N/T	N/T	10	585
grilled, 100 g	17	4	7.5	835
TOFU				
Dessert, Fruit-flavoured, Nutrisoy, 100 g	12.5	0	1	280
firm, prepared with nigari, 100 g	3	0.5	4.5	320
fried, 100 g	10.5	4	20	1135
silken, 100 g	3	0	2.5	230
tofu tempeh burgers, 100 g	N/T	N/T	9.5	730
tofu vege burgers, 100 g	N/T	N/T	9.5	730
Soy Feast, Burger Mix, 30 g	26	2	1.3	704
TOMATO				
canned in juice, 250 g	8	3	0.5	195
juice, 250 ml	9	0.5	0	195
paste, 1 tbsp	2	1	0	50
purée, 250 g	13	5	0.5	300
raw, 1 medium, 130 g	2.5	1.5	0	75
sundried, natural, 5 pieces, 10 g	5.5	1	0.5	110
sundried, in oil, drained, 3 pieces, 10 g	2.5	0.5	1.5	90
TOPPING				
caramel, Cottees, 1 tbsp	11	0	0	190
chocolate, Cottees, 1 tbsp	12.5	0	0	225
strawberry, Cottees, 1 tbsp	9	0	0	165
TORTILLA				
corn, 1, 50 g	24.5	N/T	4.5	640
wheat flour, 1, 50 g	29	N/T	4	675
TRIFLE commercial, 1 serve, 120 g	33	0.5	7	880
TRITICALE meal, 40 g	25	0	1	520
TURKEY				
baked, lean, 120 g	0	0	5	780
buffe breast, no skin, 80 g	0	0	3.5	815
buffe breast, with skin, basted, 100 g	0	0	8	610
Hamwich, Tegel, 1 slice	0	0	4	625
hindquarter, meat, 100 g	0	0	11.5	700
roast, dark meat, 100 g	0	0	4	560
roast, light meat, 100 g	0	0	1.5	560
roast, with skin, 100 g	0	0	6.5	715
Salami, Tegel, 100 g	0	0	4	625
smoked, 75 g	0	0	1	335
TURNIP peeled, boiled, 1 cup, 240 g	9	7.5	0	215
TWO FRUITS (SEE ALSO FRUIT SALAD)				
Just Fruit, Peach & Mango in Syrup, Berri, 133 g	12	1.5	0	235
Just Fruit, Sliced Peaches in Syrup, Berri, 133 g	12	1.5	0	265
Fruit Salad in Syrup, Goulburn Valley, 125 g	15	N/T	0	250
VEAL				
boneless, unspecified cut, lean, 1, 190 g	0	0	5	1185
boneless, unspecified cut, untrimmed, 1, 200 g	0	0	8	1340
cutlet, crumbed & fried, 1	0	0	5	730

TOFU & TEMPEH Made from soya beans, these are low in fat, high in calcium and excellent sources of protein for vegetarians. All soya products contain phytoestrogens, which many scientists think protect against cancers and heart disease, and may help women fight breast cancer, osteoporosis and menopausal symptoms.

FIRM TOFU This holds its shape well when cooked. It can be marinated and then fried or grilled, or cut into pieces and added to curries. Store in water in the refrigerator.

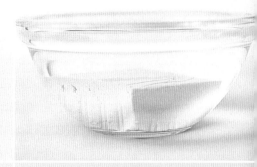

MILKEN TOFU This soft tofu can be blended and used instead of dairy products in dips, ice creams or cheesecakes. Wonderful as a simple dessert sweetened with bananas and maple syrup.

TEMPEH A fermented soya bean cake, this Indonesian food has a nutty taste and can be thinly sliced and grilled, or used in stir-fries.

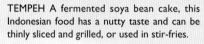
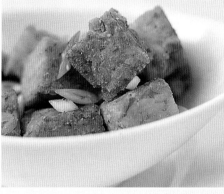

RECIPE Marinate thick slices of firm tofu in a mixture of grated ginger and soy for several hours. Fry, grill or add to a stir-fry.

FOOD	CARB	FIBRE	FAT	ENERGY
	g	g	g	kJ
forequarter steak, lean, 1, 190 g	0	0	6	1380
forequarter steak, untrimmed, 1, 200 g	0	0	10.5	1565
heart, baked, 100 g	0	0	6	760
kidney, grilled, 100 g	0	0	5.5	700
leg, lean, baked, 2 slices, 44 g	0	0	0.5	225
leg, untrimmed, baked, 2 slices, 45 g	0	0	0.5	270
leg steak, lean, fried, 1, 85 g	0	0	2.5	550
leg steak, untrimmed, fried, 1, 100 g	0	0	4	670
liver, grilled, 85 g	1.5	0	7	670
loin chop, lean, baked or grilled, 1, 50 g	0	0	1.5	305
loin chop, untrimmed, baked or grilled, 1, 55 g	0	0	2.5	370
schnitzel, fried, 1, 85 g	8.5	1	23	1205
shank, lean, simmered, 1, 80 g	0	0	2	490
shank, untrimmed, simmered, 1, 90 g	0	0	6	670
shoulder steak, lean, grilled, 1 small, 50 g	0	0	1.5	305
shoulder steak, untrimmed, grilled, 1 small, 55 g	0	0	2.5	355
VEGETABLE JUICE V8, Campbells, 250 ml	11	0	0.5	215
VEGETABLES (SEE INDIVIDUAL VEGETABLES)				
VENISON roast, 100 g	0	0	5.5	660
VINEGAR				
apple cider, 100 ml	6	0	0	60
unspecified, 100 ml	15.5	0	0	90
white, 1 tbsp	0	0	0	15
WAFFLES				
frozen, 1 square, 35 g	13.5	1	2.5	370
home-made, 1 round, 75 g	24.5	1.5	10.5	915
WATER (SEE ALSO SOFT DRINKS)				
plain mineral; soda; tap, 1 glass, 250 ml	0	0	0	0
Schweppes, average all varieties, 1 glass, 250 ml	24.5	0	0	425
WATER CHESTNUTS				
canned, drained, 40 g	3.5	1	0.5	80
raw, 5, 50 g	12	1.5	0	205
WATERCRESS raw, 1 cup, 32 g	0.5	1	0	25
WHEATGERM 1 tbsp	1.5	1	0.5	70
WITCHETTY GRUB raw, 1 large, 30 g	3.5	0	7	420
YAM baked or boiled, 100 g	30.5	2	0.5	550
YEAST				
dried, bakers, compressed, 1 sachet, 7 g	0.5	0.5	0	35
dried, brewers, 1 sachet, 7 g	0.5	2	0.5	80
YOGHURT				
acidophilus, low-fat, Honey & Strawberry, Bornhoffen, 100 ml	13	0	3	420
acidophilus, low-fat, skim milk, Attiki, 100 ml	11	0	0	235
acidophilus, plain, Attiki, 100 ml	8	0	3.3	100
Black Cherry, Yoplait, 100 ml	17	0	4	435
drinking, Apricot, Jalna, 250 ml	31	N/T	5	800
drinking, Bulla, 100 ml	13	0	1	340
drinking, Swiss Vanilla, Jalna, 250 ml	31.5	N/T	5	775

VEGETABLES Long recognised as an excellent low-fat source of dietary fibre, vitamins and minerals, vegetables are now also thought to help protect the body against some cancers. Vegetables do lose much valuable Vitamin C when cooked, so include plenty of fruit and salad in your diet too.

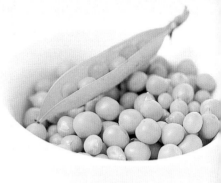

PEAS A rich source of Vitamin C, just one serving can provide half the daily requirement. Remember that freezing and boiling lose some of that Vitamin C.

BROCCOLI Extremely rich in Vitamin C, one serving contains twice the daily allowance. Boiling cuts this in half, so microwave, steam or stir-fry instead.

CORN An excellent source of Vitamin C, a good source of fibre and a moderate source of thiamin and niacin.

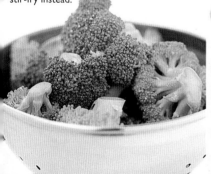

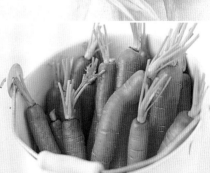

RECIPE To prepare vegetables without adding fat, steam some vegetables, drizzle with lemon juice and sprinkle with black pepper.

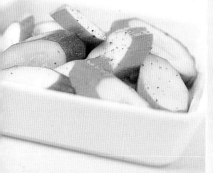

CARROT The richest plant source of beta carotene, high levels of which may protect against cancer and damage done by free radicals. Cooking carrots actually helps the body to absorb the beta carotene.

FOOD	CARB g	FIBRE g	FAT g	ENERG kJ
drinking, Vitalize, multi-vitamin, Jalna, 250 ml	24	3.5	5	585
drinking, Wild Berry, Jalna, 250 ml	31.8	N/T	5	800
frozen, Fruit Yoghurt Stick, Raspberry; Strawberry, Bulla, 65 ml	20	0	5	555
frozen, Fruit 'n Yoghurt, Bulla, 100 ml	20	0	5	555
frozen, low-fat, Baskin Robbins, 100 ml	N/T	0	3	480
frozen, low-fat, Botanica, Tea Infusions, 100 ml	22	0	0	350
frozen, no-fat, no-sugar, 1 cone	N/T	0	0	190
frozen, non-fat, Baskin Robbins, 100 ml	N/T	0	0	335
frozen, non-fat, Honey Hill Farms, 1 cone	N/T	0	0	460
frozen, reduced-fat, Honey Hill Farms, 1 cone	N/T	0	0	380
frozen, strawberry, 85 ml	N/T	0	4	535
Fruit Cocktail, Diet Lite, Nestlé, 100 ml	13	0	0.2	385
Honey, European-style, Dairy Farmers, 100 ml	11.5	0	7	555
Kiwifruit & Mango, Diet Lite, Nestlé, 100 ml	13.6	0	0.2	395
Lemon, Yoplait, 100 ml	15	0	0	345
low-fat, Berry, Diet Lite, Ski, 100 ml	15	0	1	365
low-fat, Berry Fruits, Diet Lite, Danone, 100 ml	7	0	0	180
low-fat, Fruit Salad; Blueberry; Cherry, Diet Lite, Danone, 100 ml	7	0	0	180
low-fat, passionfruit, 100 ml	16	0	0	375
low-fat, Peach, Diet Lite, Danone, 100 ml	6.5	0	0	175
low-fat, Peach & Mango, Diet Lite, Ski, 100 ml	15	0	2	815
low fat, plain, Dairy Farmers, 100 ml	6	0	0	215
low-fat, Strawberry, Diet Lite, Danone, 100 ml	6.5	0	0	175
low-fat, Summer Delights Combo, Diet Lite, Ski, 100 ml	16	0	1	390
low-fat, Vanilla, Diet Lite, Danone, 100 ml	6	0	0	170
low-fat, Vanilla Fruit & Nut Combo, Diet Lite, Ski, 100 ml	16	0	1	400
plain, biodynamic, Jalna, 100 ml	5	0	4.5	400
plain, European-style, Dairy Farmers, 100 ml	6	0	8	505
plain, Skim Milk Natural, Jalna, 100 ml	7	0	0.1	215
plain, Swiss Creamy Custard, Jalna, 100 ml	1	0	4.5	450
plain, Traditional, Dairy Farmers, 100 ml	6.5	0	3.5	325
soft serve, Colombo, 100 ml	16.5	0	0	335
soft serve, low-fat, average	N/T	0	0	335
soft serve, New Zealand Natural, 100 ml	24	0	2	595
soft serve, no cholesterol/fat-free, Gise, 100 ml	4.5	0	0	90
Strawberry Delight, Nestlé, 125 ml	20	0	4	570
Vanilla, Yoplait, 100 ml	19	0	4	480
Yakult, 65 ml	11	0	0	195
YoBaby, Banana/Vanilla, Yoplait, 100 g	N/T	0	4	450
Yogo, average all flavours, 150 g	N/T	0	5	700
YORKSHIRE PUDDING small serve, 50 g	N/T	0.5	5	435
ZUCCHINI				
green, boiled, 90 g	1.5	1.5	0.5	55
yellow, boiled, 90 g	1	1.5	0.5	70

YOGHURT The fat content in oghurt largely depends on the milk it is made from. Yoghurt is always an excellent source of calcium and B-group vitamins, and varieties made with acidophilus bacteria are increasingly taken by people wishing to keep their intestines healthy.

NATURAL YOGHURT The name says it all, it has no added flavours or colouring and is simply milk with a starter culture added. Select a low-fat variety.

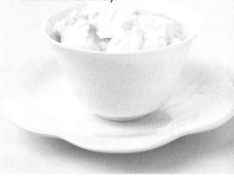

FRUIT YOGHURT Must contain at least 5% fruit. This can be juice, dried fruit, purée or pulp. Manufacturers may also add flavours, colours, sugar and thickeners.

ARTIFICIALLY SWEETENED YOGHURT Artificial sugar is added to some low-fat yoghurts to reduce the kilojoule content even further.

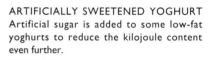

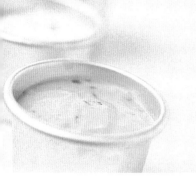

RECIPE Make your own flavoured yoghurt by adding honey, vanilla essence, puréed fruit or berries to low-fat natural yoghurt.

ACIDOPHILUS A live culture that can be added to yoghurt. There is evidence that it may help to restore levels of healthy bacteria in the gut after an infection or antibiotics.

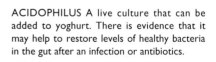

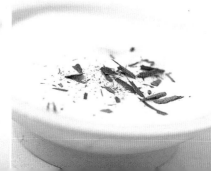

Published by Murdoch Books® a division of Murdoch Magazines Pty Ltd,
45 Jones Street, Ultimo NSW 2007

Managing Editor: Kay Halsey
Food Director: Jody Vassallo
Concept and Design: Marylouise Brammer
Additional design: Michèle Lichtenberger
Photographer: Ben Dearnley
Stylist: Kristen Anderson
Nutritionist: Thérèse Abbey
Text: Kay Halsey, Jody Vassallo
Additional text: Carolyn Lette
Nutrition Consultants: Susan Anderson, Dr Susanna Holt

CEO & Publisher: Anne Wilson
Associate Publisher/Publishing Director: Catie Ziller
General Manager: Mark Smith
International Sales Director: Mark Newman

National Library of Australia
Cataloguing-in-Publication Data
The fat, fibre and carbohydrate counter. ISBN 0 86411 837 6.
1. Food - Fat content - Tables. 2. Food - Fiber content - Tables.
3. Food - Carbohydrate content - Tables. 613.23
PRINTED IN SINGAPORE
Printed by Tien Wah Press

Australian distribution to supermarkets and newsagents by Gordon & Gotch Ltd, 68 Kingsgrove
Road, Belmore, NSW 2192. Distributed in NZ by Golden Press, a division of HarperCollins
Publishers, 31 View Road, Glenfield, PO Box 1, Auckland 1.

The Publisher wish to thank the following for their assistance in photography for this book:
The Bay Tree, Country Road Homewares, Dinosaur Designs, Empire Homewares, Jones the Grocer,
Made in Japan, Orson & Blake.

NUTRITION: The nutritional values are approximations and can be affected by biological and seasonal
variations in foods, the unknown composition of some manufactured foods and uncertainty in the
dietary database. Nutrient data given are derived from information provided by manufacturers and the
official NUTTAB95 (Diet 1) nutritional values database produced by the Australian New Zealand
Food Authority. Commonwealth of Australia copyright reproduced by permission.

IMPORTANT: Those who might be at risk from the effects of salmonella food poisoning
(the elderly, pregnant women, young children and those suffering from immune deficiency diseases)
should consult their GP with any concerns about eating raw eggs.